# Next Generation
# NCLEX-RN
# Study Guide 2023-2024

*Complete Review + 600 Test Questions and Detailed Answer Explanations (4 Full-Length Exams)*

# Table of Contents

5

# Introduction

Nursing care all over the world continues to evolve. With new research and modern tools, nursing care delivery is beginning to rise to its fullest potential. But with the advancement in technology and devices to enhance care comes a rise in expectations and demands to deliver.

Hence, more than ever before, nursing care must demand stricter standards and better expertise. This is why nursing councils and boards seek to revise and continually increase their standards for nursing licensing examinations.

This guide includes 600 practice questions with explanations and theory material to explain the most important concepts relevant to the NCLEX examination.

**How to make the most of this guide**

1. A minimum of six hours of study every week is recommended, with three to four hours studying the content material and two to three hours studying past questions.

2. Simulate examination conditions while answering the test questions, which are similar to the questions that will appear on the NCLEX-RN examination.

3. Work with friends and teams to prepare for the examination. This has been shown to be effective in helping memory retention.

Happy studying.

# Exam Information

The National Council Licensure Examination (NCLEX) examination is a licensing examination used to test nurses and determine their eligibility to practice in the United States.

The NCLEX-RN examination is for graduates with an associate's degree in nursing (ADN) or a bachelor of science in nursing (BSN).

## NCLEX Registration

1. All candidates are required to register for their professional nursing license with the state board of their choice where they intend to obtain their license.

2. Candidates must meet all the eligibility requirements of the state where they are registered to take the NCLEX-RN examinations.

3. The official testing company for the examinations is Pearson VUE, and all candidates must register with the company.

4. Successful candidates will receive an acknowledgment email from Pearson VUE once the state board confirms their eligibility to take the exams.

5. After confirmation and payment, candidates may schedule the date and time of their examination.

## Registration Fees

The registration fee for the NCLEX-RN examination is $200. There are additional charges if a candidate wants to change the exam type or nursing regulatory body after registration.

## NCLEX-RN Examination Details

The NCLEX-RN examination follows a computerized adaptive test (CAT) model.

It is a variable-length examination, meaning candidates answer anywhere from 85 to 150 questions, depending on their performance. The CAT model gives a 50% opportunity for each candidate to provide the correct answer to every question.

There are 15 pretest questions that are not scored, 52 questions from the four major areas and 18 questions from three case studies.

**How long does the exam take?**

The length of the exam varies, but candidates have up to five hours (including all breaks) to complete the examination.

The exam stops once a candidate has completed 95% accuracy.

If candidates keep answering incorrectly, they will continue to answer more questions to give them an opportunity to pass the examination until it is 95% certain that they have not passed or the five-hour time period is exhausted.

Candidates have two allotted breaks, which the computer will notify them of.

One question will be displayed at a time. The question must be answered before the test progresses. Candidates cannot go back to a previous question. It is advised not to take uninformed guesses. However, candidates should also not spend a lot of time on just one question.

Some of the terminology used in the examinations includes:

- Client: Refers to patients. Both patient and client may be used interchangeably.
- Groups: Refers to two or more clients or patients.
- Prescription: An order, intervention, remedy or treatment plan that is prescribed by an authorized health care giver.
- Exhibit: Refers to pictures, diagrams, charts or records.
- Unlicensed Assistive Personnel (UAP): Any unlicensed health care personnel who can function in a supportive role to nurses and can perform delegated tasks.

**Rules and regulations**

Candidates may NOT:

- Attempt the examination for someone else.
- Render or receive any form of assistance during the examination.
- Utilize any form of prohibited aids, such as cell phones or smart watches.
- Create any form of disturbance.
- Tamper with the computer systems used for the examination.

If any of these rules are violated, candidates risk dismissal or cancellation of results. They are also at risk of disqualification from future NCLEX examinations.

The NCLEX-RN examination is divided into four main categories:

1. Safe and Effective Care environment, which is divided into:

   a. Management of Care

   b. Safety and Infection Control

2. Health Promotion and Maintenance

3. Psychosocial Integrity

4. Physiological Integrity, which is divided into:

   a. Basic Care and Comfort

   b. Pharmacological and Parenteral Therapies

   c. Reduction of Risk Potential

   d. Physiological Adaptation

# Chapter 1: Safe and Effective Care Environment

A safe setting is required for the delivery of quality health care. That is, a safe environment for both the clients and the health personnel.

Safety in this context includes but is not limited to physical safety. For nurses, this also extends to providing quality and essential information to clients during the process of health delivery. To achieve a safe and effective care environment, nurses must master the management of care and safety and infection control.

## Management of Care

Management of care involves the provision and coordination of nursing care in such a way that the delivery of health care is safer for both the clients and the health care personnel. It entails the following components.

### Advance Directives

This term refers to legal documentation that clearly states the wishes of patients about their care should they become unable to communicate. There are several documents for this, and they include:

1. **A Living Will:** This is a document that usually contains a list of the types of treatments and health care interventions that individuals do or do not want should they no longer be able to give informed consent. It should be as specific as possible. In the event that a particular intervention or treatment is not listed in the living will, the responsibility falls to the health care proxy to make the decision. Some commonly listed interventions include CPR, invasive procedures, surgery and nasogastric intubation.
2. **Health Care Proxy/A Durable Power of Attorney for Health Care:** This document names an individual with the right to make decisions concerning health care when the patient is incapacitated.

3. **Uniform Anatomical Gift Act**: In the US, this act allows clients who are alive to agree to donate their body parts. It also allows relatives of a deceased individual to decide to donate an organ if that individual did not make the decision while alive. It includes several regulations that prevent the sale or trafficking of human body parts.

## Integrating Advance Directives into Clients' Plans of Care

In informing or educating patients about advance directives, patients must be told about self-determination.

The Self-Determination Act was passed by Congress in 1990. It gives patients the right to either accept or refuse care on admission to any health care facility. This act also allows them the right to ask for advance directives.

If an individual already has prepared advance directives, the nurse should document this in the patient's records. If the patient does not have advance directions, the individual should be educated and then allowed to make choices. Copies of patients' advance directives must be placed in their charts.

The most important thing about advance directives is to ensure they are carried out as the occasion demands. The nurse must counsel the patient, family members and members of staff who might not be familiar with advance directives.

In integrating advance directives with client care, an important document is the five wishes. The five wishes document tells health professionals and relatives the following:

- The individual who will make decisions when a patient cannot
- The types of medical interventions that a patient accepts or rejects
- How comfortable the patient wants to be during care
- How the patient wants to be treated
- What the patient wants loved ones to know

Another document that can be useful in clients' decision-making in health care is the value history. This document describes the beliefs, opinions and principles of the client. Although it is not a legal document, it is useful in determining some decisions regarding how a patient is handled and how individuals' beliefs will affect their treatment and care.

## Advocacy

Nurses are trained to be advocates for their patients. This means that when decisions are to be made for their clients, they should have the best interests of their clients at heart. Advocacy, in this sense, can take different forms. It might involve extensive education and sensitization of patients and families. It might also involve explaining diagnoses, tests or examination findings to the patients and their families. Advocacy from nurses can also involve ensuring that the plan of care is carried out safely and at the right time. Other times, advocacy can involve seeking help from other health care professionals and non-medical workers, such as spiritual advisors or social workers.

In all, the goal of advocacy is to speak on behalf of patients and always defend their rights and interests. Advocacy involves:

1.  **Being Present:** Advocacy cannot happen if the nurse is absent, especially at times that matter most. Patients spend more time with nurses and, as such, more easily open up when it comes to discussing their concerns with them. So, registered nurses (RNs) can discuss matters with doctors or other health care workers.
2.  **Listening to patients:** RNs must be patient enough to listen to the concerns and complaints of patients, even when they are not entirely correct. RNs should also pay attention to nonverbal communication. Patients might not be comfortable with the medications or interventions being prescribed. However, they might not voice their worry, and an observant nurse must take nonverbal cues to be able to address the concerns.
3.  **Discussion of specified treatment modalities with the clients and respecting whatever decisions they make:** Treatment options should be discussed in detail

with patients. Patients who understand an intervention usually cooperate more with the health care team. Therefore, the first step of advocacy is educating the clients. In doing this, the nurse should ensure that simple terms are used so that the client understands fully. Some of the things to be discussed include the treatment itself, the procedure, benefits, possible risks and side effects, personnel carrying out the procedure and alternatives to the procedure.

4. **Advocacy to staff members:** Advocacy requires updating other nursing staff members about client advocacy and how this role should be seamlessly integrated into their practice. Other information that should be provided includes the right of clients to make decisions on their health care, including accepting or rejecting medical interventions. Advocacy to other staff members should include documenting or orally communicating the client's needs to other staff members, as well as utilizing advocacy resources efficiently. For instance, this might involve getting an interpreter when a patient does not communicate in the nurse's language. It can also involve employing external resources, for instance, occupational therapists, who are non-medical health care team members.

## Delegation

In the nursing profession, delegation means a nurse transfers a responsibility or task to another nursing staff member but still retains responsibility for the outcome of the task.

To help in the appropriate delegation of responsibilities, the American Nurses Association (ANA) has created the Five Rights of Delegation.

These rights are five areas that must be clearly addressed when assigning care to other staff. They include:

- The right person
- The right task
- The right circumstances
- The right direction/communication

- The right supervision/evaluation

**The Right Task**

Is this a task to be delegated?

Not all tasks can or should be delegated. The nature of the task will determine if it can be delegated or not. Some tasks involve meeting the needs of clients who are in dynamic or unstable conditions. Here, there can be rapid changes that require quick judgment calls and higher competence. Such tasks should not be delegated.

**The Right Person**

Is this person right for the task?

An RN must assign jobs based on people's skills and knowledge. A licensed practical nurse (LPN) can be assigned tasks that involve a stable patient. Nursing assistants can be assigned tasks that have to do with the maintenance of basic hygiene. Assigning a task to the wrong professional can be dangerous and should be avoided.

**The Right Circumstances**

What is the state of the patient?

Is the patient stable or unstable? An RN should handle the care of an unstable patient. If the patient becomes stable, then the RN can delegate the task after assessing that the circumstances have changed.

**The Right Communication**

Is there a clear and detailed explanation of the task to be performed?

A task must be clearly spelled out if it is to be delegated.

**The Right Supervision**

Who will be held accountable for the outcome of this task?

Responsibility and accountability are key in the nursing profession. Suppose a supervisory role is assigned to an RN. This means the RN has oversight over members of the team, such as other RNs, LPNs and non-licensed personnel. The nurse in charge must be able to effectively assess the skills and competencies of each team member. He or she must communicate in very clear terms what each member of the team is meant to do. The RN will take responsibility for the outcome of the task.

**Organization of Workload and Time Management**

For an RN, organization and time management are nonnegotiable. This is because the management of clients in the health care setting is usually time-bound. Triaging is a very important skill that every RN must master. For some clients, it is the difference between life and death.

Some frameworks that can be used to prioritize include:

- ABCs of resuscitation — airway, breathing and cardiovascular or circulatory system. This is useful in deciding where to start attending to a patient who has undergone a cardiac arrest. However, it is important to note that the recent update has changed the sequence to CAB, meaning chest compressions come first, followed by airway and then breathing.
- Maslow's hierarchy of needs shows that the first thing to attend to is the patient's physiological needs, then safety, security, self-esteem and self-actualization.
- Agency policies as dictated by the health care facility. Different health care institutions might come up with their own specific protocols for prioritizing patients. When this is done, the nurse must follow what has been stated and look for how this can be improved upon.
- Care should be prioritized so that all clients receive their medication promptly.

In addition, a nurse should be able to clarify whether an assignment is necessary or not. A nurse should also plan work systematically, making room for changes in the status or condition of clients and priorities.

All unnecessary interruptions should be avoided, and a nurse should learn how to decline tasks from other staff members when there are higher priority needs to be addressed. Without effective organizational skills, nurses burn out quickly or spend much time and energy on less important tasks.

## Case Management

Case management in nursing involves developing, implementing and evaluating health care plans for patients. But beyond this, it is an effective method of delivering nursing care. It typically involves managing and coordinating care, identifying and effectively utilizing resources, planning referrals and connecting clients to services based on need.

### Advocating for Cost-Effective Care

As case managers, nurses ensure that the client care being delivered is of high quality, cost-effective and timely. It is the nurse's duty to explore all options with other health care team members to ensure that the patient is getting the most affordable care without a dip in quality.

There are two types of health care reimbursement: prospective and retrospective.

In the retrospective reimbursement system, health care facilities received payments for the care they rendered based on the cost, and insurance companies paid for all the services, irrespective of the costs. However, this was not sustainable as health care costs continue to rise globally.

The prospective reimbursement system came about to cut the excesses of retrospective reimbursement. Under this system, health care facilities are reimbursed a specific amount determined by the client's diagnosis. This has made more health care facilities conscious of how much is spent and makes them seek more efficient ways to cut costs and reduce the length of patient stays and resources used. Cost-effectiveness has become a priority for most health care organizations. Therefore, a nurse must understand it and utilize the least resources to produce the best results as much as possible.

**Initiate, Update and Evaluate Plan of Care**

Nurses are responsible for planning, updating and evaluating health care plans for clients. The plan that is developed for each patient must be individualized based on the patient's condition and needs. The plan must take several factors about the client into consideration, such as the diagnosis, the patient's ability to take care of him or herself, the currently prescribed treatment, actual and potential problems and more. The plan must always remain up to date based on the current needs of the client.

As case managers, nurses ensure that all the plans are carried out. This also includes the services performed by multidisciplinary team members who are not part of the nursing care team.

Nurses ensure that every patient is treated at the right level of care. They also educate clients and their families when this needs to be done, giving the reasons, the modalities and the outcomes they are trying to achieve or prevent. If it is a discharge from the health care facility, the nurse ensures that clients and their families have enough information on what to do and what is expected at home or in the community.

The models that are used in case management include:

- The ProACT model: ProACT stands for the Professionally Advanced Care Team. The Robert Wood Johnson University Hospital created this model of case management.
- Collaborative practice
- Case manager model
- Triad model of case management

## Client Rights

Clients have rights and responsibilities that must be acknowledged by health care personnel to guide their practice.

Some client rights have been examined under the self-determination act, which gives the patient the right to accept or reject care. Other rights include:

### HIPAA

The Health Insurance Portability and Accountability Act (HIPAA) protects the personal information of clients, such as name, date of birth, social security number and information on diagnosis and treatment. This act ensures that those who have access to the information are involved in the management or care of the patient.

### Patient's Bill of Rights

The Patient's Bill of Rights was adopted by the United States for the health care industry in 1998. Here are some of the key areas that every nurse should be aware of:

**1. Client information:** Every client has the right to accurate and easy-to-understand information about the plan for their health. It is important that clients know what is going on at every point in their care. If there is a communication barrier, such as a language difference, an interpreter should be provided to ensure patients clearly understand what is being done.

**2. Choice of health care provider and health care plan:** Every client has a right to choose the health care provider they want. They also have the right to choose the type of health care plan they prefer.

**3. Access to emergency services:** Every patient has the right to emergency screening and stabilization whenever they have an acute or severe condition. Patients have a right to these emergency services whenever and wherever they are needed, without authorization or financial penalties.

**4. Making treatment decisions (informed consent):** Patients have the right to know all available treatment options and decide which they prefer. They also have a right to select who can make decisions for them when they are not able to do so themselves. Patients should be clearly informed about their condition and the proposed treatment, including the benefits, risks, side effects, recovery and any other information about the procedure.

**5. Confidentiality:** Patients have a right to speak privately to their health care providers and have their information treated confidentially. They have the right to look through their medical records and request an amendment of any inaccurate information.

**6. Complaints and Appeals:** Patients have the right to a swift, fair review of any complaints they have against health care personnel or the facility.

**7. Respect:** Every client has a right to be treated with respect by health care professionals. They also have a right to be treated and attended to without discrimination from any health care worker.

**Client Responsibilities**

Client responsibilities include treating health care workers with respect, paying medical bills and other financial obligations as soon as possible, and reporting changes that are unexpected in their condition to the health care professional. They must also provide accurate information about their health, follow rules and regulations given upon admission and be responsible for their own behavior.

A nurse must ensure that clients understand their rights and that the health care professionals also understand them.

**Collaboration with Multidisciplinary Team**

Collaboration refers to the interdisciplinary interaction and cooperation between various sectors of health care. Nurses work with doctors, pharmacists, physical therapists, psychologists, social workers, nutritionists and other health care professionals to achieve optimum client care and outcome. To do this, there is a need to first:

**Identify the need for interdisciplinary conferences**

Interdisciplinary or multidisciplinary conferences involve interacting with other health care professionals involved in managing clients.

These meetings usually involve a lot of planning and the selection of an agenda, a date, a venue and a fixed time. At these meetings, nurses can serve as patient advocates, raising issues that are pertinent to client care.

They can also resolve potential conflict issues and areas of misunderstanding with other professionals. Interdisciplinary conferences are necessary for the holistic management of patients. They provide the opportunity to not only contribute to client care but also learn and observe from the perspective of other health care professionals. The goal is usually geared toward improving the delivery of client care.

In participating in interdisciplinary conferences, nurses should freely express their thoughts in a respectful manner while also listening to the points raised by other health care professionals.

**Identify significant information to report to other disciplines**

In collaboration, there must be effective and timely communication between disciplines. Interdisciplinary client care will only thrive when there is smooth communication between health care professionals.

Nurses are on the front lines and will usually detect changes in patient conditions before other health care professionals. Hence, they must be able to communicate such observations promptly and clearly.

Nurses must know the signs to look out for in a patient's condition, whether it is in vital signs or reactions to prescribed drugs. They must then channel this information to the appropriate health care personnel for immediate action.

**Review plan of care to ensure continuity across disciplines**

Nurses function as collaborators and managers of client care. Therefore, they are responsible for a continuous review of clients' care plans. Their review is to ensure that all health care professionals are doing what they should. If there is a default or deviation from the plan of care by anyone, then the nurse should point it out so that it can be corrected. It is important to note that this review has to be continuous and up to date, as the client's plan of care is being updated.

**Collaborate with multidisciplinary team members when providing client care**

Nurses collaborate with other members of the health care team to deliver quality health care. It is important that nurses maintain a high level of professionalism, good interpersonal and communication skills and sound judgment when interacting with other health care professionals.

Some other team members and their roles include:

- *RNs*: Licensed health care personnel who are trained to deliver nursing care in several health care settings can manage both stable and unstable patients in structured or unstructured environments. They are also trained to coordinate other nursing team members, such as nursing assistants and LPNs.
- *Nursing Assistants/Patient Care Technicians:* These are non-licensed assistants who help nurses to provide direct and indirect care under the direct supervision of the RN. They also help perform non-sterile procedures requiring little technical expertise, such as collecting specimens, documenting vital signs, patient movement and exercises and other patient activities required for daily living.

- *Licensed Practical Nurses*: Also licensed health care professionals, LPNs provide a wide variety of nursing care services in many different health care settings. They can perform both sterile and non-sterile procedures, and they can work with patients that are relatively stable in structured settings. They usually work under the supervision of an RN.
- *Nursing Supervisors:* Nursing supervisors are responsible for patient supervision and receiving reports from several nurses under their supervision. They then pass these reports to the nursing director.

Additional professionals include medical doctors, doctors of chiropractic medicine, dieticians, physical therapists, occupational therapists and psychologists and social workers.

**Serve as a resource to other staff**

Nurses can increase their effectiveness in collaborating with others by educating other members of the team. They can provide information about their areas of expertise and additional resources that will help other health care team members understand their roles and how to fit better into the health care team.

Medical doctors are licensed health care professionals who can provide primary care. They can also perform specialized roles, such as gynecology, cardiology, surgery and more.

Physical therapists are licensed health care personnel that provide medical interventions concerned with a patient's functional abilities. They consider factors like strength, gait and mobility and use tools like walkers and exercise routines to achieve their outcomes. They can practice in all health care settings, including the home setting.

Occupational therapists are closely related to physical therapists, but they focus more on interventions that help to restore the client to the best possible level of independence. They are concerned with functions that contribute to daily living, such as eating, bathing, wearing socks and getting dressed. Occupational therapists can work in all health care settings, including the home.

Social workers ensure that the client is appropriately moved in the continuum of care and there is no deficit after the patient is discharged. They counsel patients and can also provide psychological support. They are essential in cases of child abuse, neglect or malpractice and can provide a much-needed link and support for victims.

## Concepts of Management

Management is the process of hitting set targets by strategizing, organizing and utilizing efforts, talents and resources available. Nurses have a set target to deliver and promote high-quality care to their patients. It is their responsibility as managers to ensure that they use whatever resources are available—both human and material—to achieve this. For managerial success, nurses must:

### Identify the roles and responsibilities of health care team members

As discussed in other sections, health care personnel have different roles and responsibilities. It is the duty of the nurse to understand who plays what role and who handles what responsibilities. This way, when clients have needs, the nurse knows exactly who to call to provide the service.

If there is a need and the wrong person is called, it leads to wasted time and delays in delivering care. It also affects the schedule of the person who was mistakenly called.

Therefore, nurses should take the understanding of the roles and responsibilities of health care personnel very seriously.

### Plan overall strategies to address client problems

One important role of managers is to strategize. Client needs are important and can be overwhelming if there is no plan to attend to them. Therefore, nurses must come up with effective strategies to manage different client needs. These strategies must take into consideration the urgency of the task, as well as the personnel carrying it out.

Some of these strategies include:

- **Delegation and supervision:** As noted earlier, tasks should be delegated to personnel based on their skill level and competence.
- **The nursing process:** This includes planning, assessing, implementing and evaluating, which should all be carried out efficiently.
- **Collaboration:** Nurses do not have the training required to attend to all client problems. Therefore, it is important to always reach out to other health care team members when a need arises that is peculiar to their specialty.
- **Educating clients and staff:** Nurses occupy a pivotal role, sometimes serving as the only link between clients and other staff. This places them in an advantageous position to educate both parties. Clients might need to be educated about their condition, the prognosis, the risks, expected interventions with their benefits and side effects and more. The staff might need to be educated about the clients' rights and responsibilities and their own responsibilities toward the clients. They might also need to be educated on the patient's needs, how to solve them and how to monitor for any change in their conditions. Engagement of clients is crucial to get full cooperation. Patients tend to respond better when the health care team is more open and understanding.

**Act as liaisons between clients and others**

Advocacy has been mentioned as one of the key elements of the nursing profession. Nurses serve as advocates for the client's family members, other members of the health care team, the management of the hospital and even insurance companies. Their role as advocates is important to the managerial position they occupy.

**Manage conflict among clients and health care staff**

Conflicts or disagreements are a normal part of human interaction. They happen everywhere, and the health care setting is not exempt. Therefore, nurses must be skilled in managing conflicts among clients and health care staff.

Some of the most common causes of conflict in health care settings are:

- Disrespect
- Overworking
- Unfair distribution of roles or duties
- Ill health
- Patient loss
- Negligence
- Limited resources
- Poor remuneration
- Poor communication skills
- Different personality types

To resolve conflict, a nurse must understand the stages of conflict and conflict resolution, which include:

1. **Frustration:** The individuals involved in the conflict feel like their needs are being sidelined. It might be a need for respect, consideration of working hours, a bonus or raise or a client feeling neglected.
2. **Conceptualization:** Those affected by the conflict begin to understand what is happening and why it happened. They begin to provide logical or illogical reasons that they believe have caused the conflict.
3. **Action:** The individuals respond and act on the frustrations and conclusions that they have come to. At this point, the actions taken differ. For some, it might be lashing out in anger or physical assault. Others might just withdraw.
4. **Resolution:** At this stage, all the people involved are able to come to an amicable solution.

Lewin's four types of conflict are based on approach and avoidance concepts.

A. **Avoidance-Avoidance Conflict**: The individuals involved are not open to any of the alternatives that can lead to a resolution of the conflict. This might be because the alternatives are not appealing to either of the parties involved in the conflict.

B. **Approach-Approach Conflict:** The individuals or parties involved have more than one alternative that can resolve the conflict. This is the direct opposite of the avoidance-avoidance conflict.

C. **Approach-Avoidance Conflict:** The choices or alternatives that can resolve the conflict are not completely satisfactory to both parties. So, the choices have some positive aspects but also have some negative aspects.

D. **Double Approach-Avoidance Conflict:** The involved individuals have to choose one alternative due to its positive sides but also accept the negative sides while giving up other alternatives.

Healthy ways of resolving conflict include:

- **Collaboration and Communication:** Conflicts will be easily settled when people in a health care setting are open to cooperating and working with each other. An environment of cooperation leads to better opportunities to air grievances and differences, and it fosters better relationships among members of the team.
- **Negotiation/Compromise:** Both parties must make a move to meet in the middle. This emphasizes focusing on common goals and interests, which in this setting should be the delivery of quality care rather than focusing on personal interests and desires. It also allows individuals to explore alternatives and offer solutions to a particular problem.
- **Mediation:** This requires an impartial third party to speak individually with those involved in the conflict before bringing them together to arrive at a mutually beneficial conclusion. Many times, RNs might be required to play the role of mediators when there are conflicts.

Ineffective or unhealthy methods of conflict resolution are:

- **Avoidance:** Prolonged withdrawal and avoidance of the entire situation do not foster unity among the team, nor do they lead to needs being met.
- **Competition:** Competition is very unhealthy for the health care team when it stems from conflict. It can put patient care at risk and reduce the quality of care.
- **Accommodating others without addressing issues:** While it is good to be accommodating and considerate, issues that are important to the individual should be resolved. If a person keeps accommodating unmet needs, it will eventually affect the person's performance in the long run. It can lead to resentment and other negative behaviors.

RNs must recognize patterns of conflict. If necessary, they should step in immediately to mediate the situation and prevent a deterioration of the relationship and, ultimately, the quality of care.

## Evaluate Management Outcomes

As a manager, the goal is to always get more efficient with the use of resources. Therefore, evaluation and measurement must always be ongoing, and outcomes and results should always be measured. Were the set objectives met? Has the quality of care improved? Are the patients happy about a specific metric of care?

## Confidentiality/Information Security

HIPAA provides protection of health information for individuals in the United States. It also gives patients the right to know what can or can't be done with their health information.

But this rule also balances the confidentiality of patient information with necessary disclosure for the provision of quality health care or insurance or reimbursement.

The confidentiality that HIPAA mandates health care workers to keep is not just limited to written information. It also covers electronic and online information about a patient's health status and must not be shared with anyone except those providing medical care and those the patient has documented in writing.

**Maintaining client confidentiality and privacy**

HIPAA provides legal protection for patients' medical records and limits the sharing of information by whatever means to only those who need to know. The "need to know" population comprises those who need the medical information of the patient in order to render direct or indirect patient care. Direct patient care refers to those who directly provide a form of care to the patient, such as nurses, physical therapists, doctors and others. Indirect care covers those who do not directly provide a form of care but still have a role to play in patient care, such as insurance providers, directors of nursing and more.

Another aspect of maintaining client privacy is the privacy given to them during visits and conversations with their families or guests.

In addition to HIPAA, health care facilities and institutions usually have their own regulations that help protect client privacy. Nurses should maintain these regulations at all times. Failure to do so can make a nurse liable for legal actions.

**Assess staff member and client understanding of confidentiality requirements**

One of the most effective ways to assess staff members' understanding of confidentiality requirements is by observation. As they carry out their daily routines, they observe the manner in which they discuss patients and the way they use online medical records. Do they log out after finishing their task? Are they casual about opening client information anywhere? Do they talk about their patients online or post images of their patients on social media?

You can also assess clients' understanding of client rights on confidentiality by observation. A client who asks for information about another client's case is unlikely to understand confidentiality in his or her own health care.

**Intervene appropriately when staff members have breached confidentiality**

A nurse is an advocate for the rights of the patient and when any of these rights are breached, a nurse must be able to advocate for correction immediately.

## Continuity of Care

Continuity of care refers to the seamless movement of a patient from one section to another in the same health care facility or from one health care facility to another. This continuity of care can be from a higher to a lower level of intensity of care or vice versa. It can be from a primary to a secondary or tertiary health care facility. The patient can also be discharged from the health care facility.

All these constitute transitions, which are referred to as continuity of care. At every level, care must be ongoing. The only difference is the type and intensity of care.

To ensure that this process is seamless, nurses have a major role to play in organization, communication and collaboration.

**Provide and receive a handoff of care report on assigned clients**

It is essential to ensure a seamless transfer of patients at the end of shifts. The smooth handover of patients' forms is one of the basic elements of nursing care. This is because patient care is severely affected when a transfer is not seamless. It can affect medication plans, timing and the overall quality of care. Hence, nurses must take this aspect of care seriously and go over every detail during the handover.

At the very minimum, reports should include the name of patients, the attending doctor's name, the admission date and the diagnosis made. They should also include the completed and uncompleted tasks, care priorities, critical information about the health status of the patient, how responsive the patient has been to treatment, fluid input/output, observed unusual incidents, any special interventions, blood transfusion and if there was an adverse reaction, consults/referrals, any alteration in the care plan or doctor's orders.

Highlighting all these might be cumbersome and difficult to remember during a handover. So, bodies like The Joint Commission on the Accreditation of Health Care Organizations have come up with standardized handoff reports. They include:

- SBAR (Situation, Background, Assessment, Recommendations)
- ISBAR (Introduction, Situation, Background, Assessment, Recommendation)
- BATON (Background, Actions, Timing, Ownership, Next)
- IPASS (Introduction, Patient, Assessment, Situation, Safety Concerns)
- The five P's (Patient, Plan, Purpose, Problems, Precautions).

All these provide a way of reporting essential information that must be passed on to the next nurse.

## Use documents to record and communicate client information

Documenting is pivotal to client care. In fact, some health care workers claim what is not documented is not done. A nurse must have a strong culture of documenting things. This is very important in the continuum of care. It provides a basis for assessment since what has been done and what is left to be done is clearly stated.

Different health care facilities have documents that they use as admission forms, vitals charts, fluid input and output forms, referral forms, discharge forms and more.

It is the nurse's responsibility to understand the guidelines for each form.

## Use approved terminology when documenting care

Another critical area to pay attention to is the terminology used in documentation. Sometimes what is written is the only record available for health care. Therefore, great care must be taken to determine how something is written.

Health care facilities must have a list of permitted abbreviations and what they stand for to avoid misunderstandings and miscommunications. There should also be a list of prohibited abbreviations so that these are not used during documentation.

**Perform procedures necessary to safely admit, transfer and/or discharge a client**

Continuity of care basically involves admission, transfer, discharge and referral of patients.

Admission refers to the first initial client contact, which results in a person entering the ward or health care facility. A transfer involves moving a patient from one section of the same health care facility to another. A discharge is a termination of care and services rendered on admission into health care. However, other services may continue. For instance, a patient might be discharged from the ward of a health care facility to the clinic of the same facility for regular check-ups or monitoring. A patient might also be discharged to another facility for follow-up.

Admission into a facility or ward will usually require that the client is thoroughly assessed, including the reasons for admission or transfer to another receiving section of the facility. It should involve detailed notes or reports from the transferring section or facility.

The nurse should educate the patient on the regulations of the health care section or facility, including the visiting hours, number of guests allowed, rules about privacy and confidentiality, use of restrooms and more.

On discharge, there should be effective communication between the discharging section or facility and receiving section or facility. There should be adequate documentation about the status of the patient on admission and then status on delivery, noting the important changes that necessitated a discharge.

Other necessary documents from health care personnel should also be reviewed.

**Follow up on unresolved issues regarding client care**

Laboratory results and scans should all be followed up so that results are not missed. Nurses should take follow-up seriously at all times, and even if they are not able to resolve issues in their shift, they can communicate to the next nurse on shift or escalate the matter to higher authorities to be addressed.

**Establishing Priorities**

Establishing priorities is a skill every nurse must master.

**Apply knowledge of pathophysiology when establishing priorities for interventions with multiple clients**

When handling multiple clients, the importance of evidence-based care cannot be overemphasized. The nurse should be familiar with disease and injury patterns and changes.

The knowledge of pathophysiology should guide the delivery of care. A nurse should understand changes that can occur, whether negative or positive, and when they are most likely to occur. These changes are either physiological or psychological, and they determine how health interventions will be carried out.

For instance, in attending to different clients with complaints in an emergency room, the nurse should bear in mind that patients who present with breathing difficulties should be attended to before people with minor cuts or bruises. And a patient who is on the verge of entering into shock will need swift attention compared to a patient who has the flu.

Checking for abnormal pulse rates, increased blood pressure, respiratory problems or other diagnostic test values is also important.

In general, when a patient presents with certain complaints, knowledge of disease trends will aid in swift assessment, diagnosis and planning of the client's care as necessary.

**Prioritize the delivery of client care based on acuity**

In delivering quality care to a patient, accuracy is vital in determining what comes first. Clients should be managed after identifying and differentiating biological needs from social needs.

For instance, in the admission of three clients into the ward, Client A is a postoperative patient with arrhythmia and uncontrolled pain. Client B is a new patient transferred to the ward from the outpatient clinic with stable vital signs. Client C is a patient with a chest tube and on blood transfusion.

Prioritizing is based on the right knowledge, direct observation, vital assessment ratings and tools within the health care practice.

Acuity helps in the critical thinking process and also helps to identify severe conditions that should take precedence in nursing interventions.

**Evaluate plan of care for multiple clients and revise plan of care as needed**

Evaluation is significant in nursing interventions. It finalizes the basis for acuity in client care. This first includes a thorough review of all the plans of care and treatment before the nurse can determine if new care plans are to be implemented.

Although evaluation is done at the end of the nursing process, it must not be overlooked because it implies whether an intervention is successful. Also, to perform proper evaluation, documentation must have taken place consistently throughout the patient's stay in the health facility.

In assessing and diagnosing multiple clients, which will eventually lead to continuity of care, it is important to analyze if all decisions made by the nurse in prioritizing care helped in the recovery.

## Ethical Practice

### Recognize and report ethical dilemmas

Ethical dilemmas cannot be avoided in the nursing practice. However, they can be duly recognized and reported while classifying each into the appropriate categories. Many of these issues are centered on protecting the rights of a patient, planning for palliative care, confidentiality, privacy and involving clients in decision-making.

For instance, a patient in severe pain due to a femoral fracture and who has had an ORIF (Open Reduction and Internal Fixation) procedure is likely to request opioids or narcotics. This could pose a serious challenge to the nurse's profession and adherence to ethical standards, even while trying to serve the client's best interests.

Therefore, the nurse should be ready to report the situation to a superior to advocate for the patient's needs.

Also, in end-of-life scenarios, the nurse should discuss the prognosis of the illness before a decision is made in the interest of the patient. Here, detailed evidence of full disclosure should be documented.

Another example is the case study of a parent who refuses immunization for her child. No matter how attached the nurse is to the situation, after proper health education has been given to a parent who still refuses the vaccine, it is essential to report the entire process. This is done by documenting the education provided as well as a valid declaration of refusal despite all potential risks stated.

### Inform client and staff members of ethical issues affecting client care

There should be an avenue to convey the right information about a health issue to a client or colleagues to ensure proper care planning, review and continuity of care.

**Practice in a manner consistent with the nurses' code of ethics**

The nurses' code of ethics concerns behavior that is morally right for a nurse in professional situations. Therefore, the decision to elevate the standard of the profession while seeking to promote health care is vital.

The purpose of the code of ethics is to provide a framework for decision-making.

Various countries have nursing codes of ethics, such as the American Nursing Association (ANA), Royal College of Nursing (RCN) or the International Council of Nurses (ICN), with a worldwide representation of professional nurse associations.

The fundamental responsibility of the nurse is to prevent illness, promote health, restore health and alleviate suffering. Clients in need of nursing care should receive it without bias and with respect for life, human rights and dignity.

This care should be done while also maintaining a cooperative relationship with colleagues in the profession and other medical practitioners in the field.

**Evaluate outcomes of interventions to promote ethical practice**

The code of ethics is revised from time to time to include any developments or updates that take place. This includes changes in technology, the community, expansion of nursing practice into advanced practice roles, research, education, health policy and administration.

**Information Technology**

**Receive, verify and implement health care provider orders**

One of the main obligations of the nurse to the client is to ensure that health care orders are accurately received and reported.

Nurses receive orders through diverse outputs. This could be through document format, electronic format or other means.

It is vital that when these orders are received, the nurse checks for errors in the patient's age, allergies, diagnosis, medications and routes of administration and verifies the right date of admission.

After receiving orders, the nurse is expected to verify them by asking for confirmation or clarity from health care providers. Inputting the information should be done with continuity of care in mind. Only then can the implementation of the orders take place.

**Apply knowledge of facility regulations when accessing client records**

All information about a client should be handled in line with the facility guidelines, even while handing it over to other colleagues or medical practitioners.

There should be no discussions with individuals who are not directly involved in clients' care.

Thus, personal privacy, including privacy during visits and during conversations, as well as securing electronic records with passwords, is highly recommended.

**Access data for clients through online databases and journals**

Obtaining information about clients' care through online databases helps to provide a valid basis for the treatment and management of illnesses.

The nurse reviews a patient with the aid of a database to gain insight into better professional care, diagnostic procedures, clinical reports and medication use.

Also, online databases and journals contain information and resources that are derived from evidence-based activities. Through this, the nurse gains access to scientific data by combining the best knowledge available from evidence, clinical experiences and the patients' values.

**Enter computer documentation accurately, completely and promptly**

In the process of entering computer documentation, there is a need for clarity and precision. The nurse is expected to enter all vital information about a patient in an organized format from the time of admission until discharge.

This documentation is necessary to identify nursing interventions that have been provided to patients and to show patient progress during hospitalization. Other changes in patterns of care or administration should be documented as well.

**Utilize resources to promote quality client care (evidence-based research, information technology, policies and procedures)**

Utilizing resources to improve health care, identify inefficiency and promote performance assessment is vital.

Nurses make use of strategies and tools such as electronic records and organizational procedures that will help improve the quality of care rendered.

These resources help in measuring progress and evaluating the validity and reliability of the measures and sources of data received.

## Legal Rights and Responsibilities

Nursing care comes with legal responsibilities.

**Identify legal issues affecting the clients**

Legal issues that affect clients are centered on the rights of a patient to be protected by the nurse and informed about any procedure to be carried out. For instance, in the case of a client who has refused treatment or demands discharge against medical advice, proper education is key, as well as documentation of evidence. A nurse is expected to act in the best interest of the patient, per the principle of beneficence.

**Identify and manage client valuables according to facility/agency policy**

Upon discharge or termination of care, client valuables will be returned and must not be misplaced or mixed up. All items kept should be documented, with adequate descriptions and signatures of both parties involved.

**Recognize limitations of self and others and utilize resources**

The legal system requires nurses to utilize resources provided to care for clients and not accept roles that do not fulfill nursing responsibilities.

For example, a client admitted into the hospital has a three-month-old baby. The client's husband pleads for the nurse to help care for the baby.

In this situation, the nurse can politely decline and refer the husband to a pediatric clinic. Legally, since the baby was not admitted along with the mother, the nurse cannot provide it with care.

The nurse should document that education was given about the client's baby's health and the baby was referred to the pediatric unit for further care.

**Review facility policy and legal considerations before agreeing to serve as an interpreter for the staff or primary health care provider**

Clients who don't speak English may ask for translators or interpreters.

Nurses must understand all laws and regulations pertaining to interpreting. Some states allow sign language interpretation for the deaf as well as Braille use for the blind.

For facilities funded by the federal government, clients have the right to an interpreter and should not be refused one. Documenting that the client understood all information is important to have with the date, time, name and signature appended.

**Educate clients and staff on legal issues**

A framework is usually set by professional bodies on ethical standards to prevent legal issues. The nursing officer is responsible for educating clients on the consequences of refusing care either for themselves or family members, which must be reported and documented.

Likewise, overall legal reviews are made to set a guide for nursing staff and other medical practitioners. This will help to identify what is expected of caregivers and provide an understanding of legal issues that could affect services neglected or rendered.

**Report client conditions as required by law**

The condition in which a client has been admitted, and the circumstances surrounding incidents such as abuse, gunshot wounds, road accidents, burns, harmful diseases or cases of food poisoning should be reported by law.

It is in the best interest of the nurse to gather all information needed and relay it to the legal authorities. Then, a detailed investigation can be carried out in the best interest of the client, which is the focus of the nurse.

In the situation of a client who was involved in a fight or abused by a partner, information may be provided by an eyewitness, which should be well documented in clear terms.

Failure to report issues of rape or sexual assault, theft and injury could be termed negligence on the part of the nurse.

**Provide care within the legal scope of practice**

All care provided by the nurse should be within the legal scope of practice. All care rendered should be properly documented. Informed consent should be received, and the confidentiality of the patient should be respected.

It is not the role of a nurse to handle certain laboratory tests, although some facilities allow the nurse to conduct urine tests, glucose level checks and more.

## Performance Improvement (Quality Improvement)

Performance improvement focuses on enhancing and improving the quality and outcomes of care, increasing the efficiency of patient care while reducing costs, risks and liabilities. Some of the activities involved in performance improvement include:

- Identifying the improvement opportunity
- Convening a team to carry out the quality improvement
- Data collection and analysis
- Joint exploration of process under study
- Elimination of variances that can negatively affect patient care

## Define performance improvement/quality assurance activities

Some important terms in understanding performance improvement are:

- **The culture of safety:** Any health care organization must have an established culture of safety, which must run from the top echelon of the organization to the employees.
- **A blameless environment:** A blame-free environment is required for conducting performance improvement. A blameless environment is one where problems and mistakes are seen as opportunities for improvement. In this type of environment, the focus is not on the individual who made a mistake but on the different ways to improve the processes and workflow and make it fail-proof.
- **Root cause analysis:** Very closely related to a blame-free environment is the root cause analysis, which focuses on the cause of the problem. It is a process utilized in performance improvement activities focusing on the "why" rather than the "who." The root cause analysis focuses on the points of risk and vulnerability which are likely to result in errors in the health care organization. Root cause analysis can only be carried out in a blameless environment.

40

- **Sentinel events:** A sentinel event refers to an incident or accident that led to or could potentially cause harm to a client. Examples of such events include the suicide of a client, abduction of infants, falls, wrong procedures performed and adverse drug reactions, among others.
- **Variance tracking:** This involves identifying and analyzing variances that are integral to performance improvement. Variances can be either specific or random. Random variances occur when the process under study is faulty and vulnerable to human error. They occur at sporadic or unpredictable times. A specific variance occurs whenever the faulty process is carried out. It is predictable and usually occurs when a specific part of the process is faulty or vulnerable to human error.

**Performance and Quality Indicators**

Quality indicators are divided into core and outcome measures.

Core measures refer to standard measurements of quality. They are developed by the JCAHO and evaluate values like the population of clients, specific diseases and organizational measures.

Outcome measures focus on the outcomes of care. They focus on the results that are obtained after a patient has received health care. They include MRSA infection rates, lengths of stay, effectiveness of fall prevention and morbidity rates.

Risk management is concerned with reducing and eliminating dangers and health care hazards that can result in a liability to the company. Examples of these are infant abduction, patient falls and medication errors. These risks can be identified and eliminated using root cause analysis.

**Participate in performance improvement projects and quality improvement processes**

RNs may participate in performance improvement activities. For effectiveness, these activities are usually carried out in groups. It is expedient that nurses are found to be dependable, committed, adaptable and disciplined team members. They should also communicate well and add value at whatever points they can.

Performance improvement activities can be done through several methods, some of which include:

- The PDCA cycle, which involves Planning, Doing, Checking and Acting.

- The Six Sigma method, which involves problem definition, measuring, analysis of data, improvements to make and control.

- The method de jour, which is currently the most popular.

All these methods have some features that are common to all, which include:

- Problem definition

- Relevant data collection

- Analysis of collected data

- Root cause analysis

- Generating possible solutions or alternatives

- Narrowing down to a solution or alternative with the greatest feasibility and highest chance of success

- Evaluation of the effectiveness of the implemented solution

**Report identified client care issues to appropriate personnel**

Whenever there is an issue surrounding client care, nurses must promptly report it to the supervising nurse or whoever oversees the health care facility.

Most health care facilities have a structure for reporting client issues that is composed of:

- Channels of verbal communication through which concerns are orally communicated.

- Formal documents for reporting client concerns.

- Names and departments in charge of receiving such concerns.

When nurses report patient care problems accurately and promptly, they ensure proper evaluation to detect the root cause of problems and prevent their reoccurrence.

**Utilize research and other references for performance improvement actions**

Performance improvement activities require some research to see what is being done by other health care facilities and to stay updated with current practices. Some resources that a nurse can utilize for reference and research purposes include published articles, research studies, standards of care and practice, published evidence-based practices, relevant law and ethical codes. A nurse should serve as a source of improvement resources for the health care institution.

**Evaluate the impact of performance improvement measures on client care and resource use**

After all is said and done, the impact of performance improvement activities should be measured. There are several ways to do this, which include:

- Comparing the data before and after the corrective action.
- Evaluating if the resulting action plans were effective in terms of increasing client safety, efficiency, prompt delivery of care or decreasing costs or the number of patients involved in accidents or adverse events.
- Determining if the action plans were effective in the elimination of waste and efficient use of resources at the appropriate level of care.

## Referrals

### Assess the need for referrals and obtain necessary orders

Referrals are contacts that a nurse or other health care team members initiate so that the client's needs can be appropriately catered for at the required level of care and in the right setting.

It is the nurse's responsibility to ascertain when a referral becomes necessary and provide all the needed documentation and orders to ensure the process is seamless.

### Assessing the client

In referring, the first step is to assess the client's needs and if the nursing staff and other health care professionals can adequately meet the need. If a referral is necessary, then there should also be a reason for the referral. The reason could be due to a present problem that the client is facing. The reason can also be due to a potential problem that a client could face based on their present condition.

### Obtaining necessary orders

Once a need for referral is recognized, the RN should make contact with the appropriate external resource that can meet the need of the client. This external resource can be a physical therapist or even a clergy member who can offer the required help to the client.

A nurse must be able to recognize the appropriate resources for common referral needs.

Examples are:

- Individuals who perpetrate abuse might need anger management programs.
- Uninsured clients might require social workers.
- Self-help groups in the community can be suggested for those who battle addiction or other mental health conditions.

- Shelters and housing can be recommended for clients who might be victims of abuse.
- Elderly day care can be suggested for older patients.

## Safety and Infection Control

Maintaining a safe and effective care environment is incomplete without placing proper safety and infection control measures in place. These measures ensure that clients, as well as health care personnel, are protected from potential health and environmental hazards.

### Accident/Error/Injury Prevention

Preventive measures are highly important in safety and infection control. From accidents to injuries and administrative errors, there are many unfavorable incidents nurses can prevent from either occurring or escalating when they follow the right procedures during health care administration.

Preventive measures are extensive, and they begin even before a patient is admitted. They include setting up the right environment for effective patient care, planning for emergencies, anticipating and working to eliminate errors and ensuring patient-specific risk factors as soon as a patient is admitted.

#### *Assess the Client for Allergies and Intervene as Needed*

Patients may show symptoms of allergies when exposed to certain materials. Common allergies include medication and food allergies, latex reactions and other reactions to materials and substances in the air.

Before administering care, patients should be assessed for existing allergies. This ensures only the safest procedures, equipment and materials are utilized for individual patient care.

Nurses must also be able to recognize early signs of allergic reactions and what triggers they may be associated with. Certain reactions, known as anaphylactic reactions, can be life-threatening. It is therefore important that nurses are able to immediately recognize these reactions and take necessary precautions.

Common allergy symptoms include but are not limited to swelling, numbness, itching or tingling at the exposure point, breathing difficulties, rashes or bumps, hypotension and tachycardia. Swelling, numbness or tingling sensations around the lips, mouth or tongue usually indicate serious allergic reactions.

Nurses must also be aware of the appropriate intervention for each allergic reaction. Once an allergy is detected, it must be properly attended to and the trigger must be removed immediately. Every allergic reaction must be documented in order to inform future health care measures.

### Assess Client Care Environment

The client care environment refers to the physical and social setting in which nursing care is provided. Assessing the client care environment involves considering factors such as safety, comfort, privacy and cultural sensitivity.

Safety is a priority, and nurses should ensure that health care environments are continually kept safe from threats and potential hazards. The environment must be regulated to minimize falls and other injuries. Materials and equipment used should be sterile or properly disinfected before reuse, and all allergens must be removed. The environment should also be checked for factors that can trigger self-harm or aggression in patients.

The client-care environment must be assessed for physical and emotional comfortability. Bedding and other facilities provided should be comfortable for each patient's unique condition. Privacy must be catered to, and the care environment should support individual patient confidentiality.

Note that assessing the client care environment is a process that needs to be done continuously—before patients are admitted, while they are in the facility and after they've been discharged.

### Determine Client and Staff Member Knowledge of Safety Procedures

Both clients and health care workers should be assessed for their knowledge of the right safety procedures for each situation. This can be done by conducting surveys in the form of questionnaires, group discussions and one-on-one interactions.

Staff members should be adequately trained to attend to patients with safety and infection control in mind. All staff members must be aware and updated on policies and procedures for ensuring safety and should be continuously trained to manage situations effectively.

On the other hand, clients should be properly guided on how to deal with their unique situations and avoid escalations. Educational materials can be developed in simple and accessible forms for patients, caregivers, family members and friends.

### Identify Factors that Influence Accident and Injury Prevention

Some situations can serve as risk factors for the occurrence of accidents and injuries. These include factors like the patient's developmental stage, lifestyle and mental health status. Children and the elderly are more prone to accidents and injuries than adults, while the mental health status of some patients can make them prone to self-inflicted injuries.

Nurses should remain aware of these factors and work to ensure they do not trigger patient accidents.

### Identify Deficits that May Impede Client Safety

Hearing, sensing and perception deficits must be identified and considered when administering care to patients. Patients with deficits might require care in special environments, with close supervision, in order to prevent accidents. Patients who use assistive equipment must be put in ideal environments and properly monitored to ensure their assistive devices do not become potential risk factors.

### Identify and Verify Orders for Treatments that may Contribute to Accident or Injury

Certain treatment measures and procedures, aside from medication, may contribute to accidents, injuries and other negative health escalations in patients. Nurses can check this by monitoring the patient's conditions to identify treatment measures that can become risks and determine the best procedures for treatment.

Each patient's medical history should be reviewed for information such as underlying health conditions, allergies and other adverse reactions that can be triggered by certain treatments. All new findings should be properly documented to guide future health care measures.

### Identify and Facilitate the Correct Use of Infant and Child Car Seats

Car seat laws and requirements for infants and children can vary by state. However, most laws require that infants and toddlers be strapped in car seats until a child is 4'9" or 80 pounds. Nurses must stay aware of specific requirements in their states and should educate parents and guardians on the proper use of car seats and other safety measures for children.

### Promote Staff Safety

The process of ensuring a safe and secure environment for health care is not complete without looking out for the safety of staff members. Without the right measures, staff members can become potential safety and infection threats to patients and their families and vice versa.

Here are a few things that can be done to promote staff safety:

**Provide Education and Training:** Providing education and training to staff members on safety procedures, including emergency codes, infection control and workplace violence prevention, is highly important not just for the safety of patients but also for the staff's own safety and well-being.

**Provide Personal Protective Equipment (PPE):** Providing staff members with appropriate PPE, such as gloves, gowns, masks and goggles, ensures maximum protection from infectious and other hazardous materials. Not only should these provisions be made available, but staff members should be trained on how to properly wear, remove, dispose of or prepare PPE for reuse.

**Create a Safe and Ideal Work Environment:** All equipment should be properly maintained and in good working order. Hazards and obstacles should be removed, and adequate lighting should be provided in all areas of the health care facility.

**Encourage Staff Communication:** Staff members should be encouraged to communicate any safety concerns they may have, such as hazards in the work environment or concerns about patient behavior. There should be an open and supportive environment that makes staff members feel comfortable speaking up.

*Provide Clients with Appropriate Methods to Signal Staff Members*

Patients should be provided with the right methods for signaling staff members and ensuring they can communicate their needs and receive assistance when necessary.

Some of the key methods for signaling staff members are:

- Call bells

- Communication boards

- Intercom systems

- Bedside monitors

- Personal Emergency Response Systems (PERS)

### *Protect Client from Injury*

Patients have a high chance of exposure to injuries in the health care environment. Therefore, it is important for nurses to watch out for these risk factors, provide options for mitigating them and educate clients on how to request assistance or avoid falls and other kinds of injuries.

Appropriate care workers and other staff workers should be positioned in key locations like bathrooms and showers, and families and friends should be enlightened on important safety measures.

The health care environment should be designed to minimize risk factors for falls and injuries. This includes providing handrails in bathrooms and showers, setting up guard rails on patients' beds, providing appropriate lighting, minimizing room and floor clutter, removing hazardous substances, ensuring that all equipment is in good working order and setting up alarms so patients can alert health care workers in the event of a fall or any other type of injury.

Assistive devices should be recommended and provided for those who need them. Clients should be trained on how to install, uninstall and properly use these devices. Lastly, medication should be administered safely and professionally. Nurses should check medication orders for accuracy, verify medication dosages and monitor clients for potential side effects.

### *Review Necessary Modifications with Clients to Reduce Stress on Specific Muscle or Skeletal Groups*

Due to extended periods of immobility, patients may begin to experience stress on specific muscle or skeletal groups. Nurses can help facilitate stress reduction in their clients and make them more comfortable by encouraging them to perform routine muscular and skeletal exercises such as stretching and frequently changing positions.

Patients who are unable to change their positions by themselves should be turned every two hours. Such clients should also be assisted in performing stretching exercises so the strength and mobility of the body can be preserved.

Clients and their caregivers should be enlightened on the best positions and bodily alignments to maintain. These include the Sim's or semi-prone position, the prone position, the Fowler's position, the lateral position and the dorsal recumbent position. They should also be taught how to use supports like pillows, wedges and bolsters.

### Implement Seizure Precautions for At-Risk Clients

Nurses should implement seizure precautions for patients who are at risk. These precautions include identifying and removing environmental triggers, removing dangerous materials patients can latch on to during seizures, lowering the patient's bed to the lowest setting or placing the mattress on the ground, using beds with padded side rails and having oxygen and suction equipment at the patient's bedside at all times.

Intervention procedures during a seizure include helping the patient into a side-lying position and administering oxygen in the event of difficulty breathing.

### Make Appropriate Room Assignments for Cognitively Impaired Clients

Cognitively impaired clients should be admitted to rooms that allow for close monitoring. The rooms must be designed to prevent accidents and injuries to patients and ensure ease of access to treatment and medical observations.

### Properly Identify Clients when Providing Care

It is important to properly identify clients when providing care to avoid errors such as mismatched prescriptions, which can be life-threatening.

It is recommended to have at least two distinct identifiers aside from the room number of clients. Room numbers in themselves should not be used as unique identifiers.

Rather, nurses should consider using patients' full names, complete dates of birth and other unique identification measures.

Nurses should also stay mindful of patients who are at higher risk of identification errors. These include patients who cannot communicate in English, cognitively impaired patients and patients who have similar names as other registered patients.

### *Verify Appropriateness and Accuracy of a Treatment Order*

Nurses must never be in a hurry or careless about administering treatment. They should verify the appropriateness and accuracy of each treatment order, especially when they appear out of place or questionable. Nurses should reach out to the health care personnel who have prescribed such treatments or procedures for proper verification. To be successful at this, nurses must have an awareness of what medication and prescriptions are appropriate for each patient based on factors like age, stage of disease and more.

### Emergency Response Plan

The Joint Commission requires every health care facility to have an emergency response plan. This, in turn, demands every staff member understand and be properly drilled on how to handle emergency situations effectively.

### *Identify Nursing Roles in Disaster Planning*

Nurses must be prepared to handle all kinds of emergencies, including those that occur within the confines of medical facilities, such as fire hazards, workplace violence, radiation contamination, building collapse and other utility failures. These are known as internal disasters. They must also be prepared to handle emergencies within or outside their communities, such as disease outbreaks, fires, wars, natural disasters and other incidents that could result in mass casualties. These are known as external disasters.

The role of a nurse in the face of disaster and other emergencies may vary, but it will include attending to affected casualties and preventing the escalation of harm to patients and staff. To do this, nurses may be assigned to perform triage, administer treatment, track patient health and discharge patients as soon as they can be discharged to provide room for more casualties.

During triage, nurses should identify patients' situations from most critical to least critical and determine what interventions each patient needs. Critical situations should be attended to first, and in situations of equipment and bed shortages, non-critical patients may be treated and discharged immediately.

In certain disasters, nurses will teach volunteers basic first aid and caregiving principles to ease the burden of professional medical staff members while ensuring they can focus on the most critical situations.

The primary role of a nurse in the face of disaster is to ensure patients are not just treated but also kept safe from further harm.

### Determine which Clients to Recommend for Discharge in a Disaster Situation

During disasters with mass casualties, it is common to have many patients awaiting treatment. Nurses should use critical thinking and their knowledge of triage to ensure all patients are attended to, even in such difficult situations.

Priorities should be set to determine patients who should be recommended for quick discharge or relocation, while the most critical patients should be attended to first.

Ambulatory clients who require little-to-no assistance should be the first to be discharged after they have been treated, given prescriptions and received other necessary instructions. Unstable patients are high priority and are, therefore, not candidates for discharge. Stable patients who still require medical care and assistance should also be considered for admission into the facility. In the event of a lack of space, however, they may be carefully relocated to other available facilities while being strictly monitored.

*Use Clinical Decision-Making/Critical Thinking for Emergency Response Plan*

All RNs must be aware of how their decisions can impact the well-being of patients, whether positively or negatively. They must deploy critical thinking and sound decision-making skills at all times, but most especially in the face of emergency situations.

*Participate in Emergency Planning and Response*

Nurses are instrumental in participating in emergency planning and implementing response plans in the face of such emergencies. To make effective plans, nurses must stay aware of their roles in accordance with the policies applicable in their locality.

These policies will inform nurses of how they can get involved in planning and preparing for emergencies. Nurses should engage in drill sessions and practices that mimic common emergency situations, such as fire hazards, building collapse, terrorist attacks, heart attacks and other accidents that can occur within or outside the health care environment.

Nurses must stay up to date with the appropriate emergency protocols for each situation, including evacuation procedures and communication systems. Communication is an important component of a successful emergency response plan. Each health care organization may have prescribed procedures for communication in different emergency situations. Nevertheless, nurses should be able to use intuition to discern and plan ahead for the most effective ways to communicate during emergencies in order to avoid further risks.

Many organizations utilize code names to quickly and efficiently communicate different emergency situations. These codes serve as a standardized method of alerting staff and initiating appropriate responses. Here are a few examples:

- Code Blue: This code is commonly used to indicate a cardiac arrest or a medical emergency requiring immediate resuscitation.
- Code Red: This code is typically used to signify a fire or the presence of smoke within the facility, prompting immediate evacuation and fire response protocols.

- Code Orange: When there is a chemical spill or release of hazardous materials, Code Orange is often used to alert personnel and initiate appropriate containment and decontamination procedures.
- Code Pink: This code is commonly associated with infant abduction or the disappearance of a newborn, triggering a coordinated effort to locate and ensure the safety of the infant.
- Code Gray: Used for severe weather conditions such as hurricanes, cyclones or other intense storms, Code Gray prompts preparedness measures and response protocols to ensure the safety of individuals in the affected area. Other organizations may use Code Gray to refer to assault instead of severe weather conditions.

## *Participate in Disaster Planning Activities/Drills*

RNs are expected to participate in workshops and drills for planning emergency responses in the face of disasters. These workshops are designed to inform, train and encourage collaboration with other health care providers during emergencies.

## Ergonomic Principles

## *Use Ergonomic Principles when Providing Care*

Nurses should consider ergonomic principles and body mechanics when providing care to clients and helping them use assistive devices. All devices, facilities and equipment should allow patients, their caregivers and other health care workers to safely move from one point to another or move distinct body parts.

Ergonomic principles should be observed when:

- Moving patients from one point to the other on stretchers and wheelchairs.

- Helping patients maintain a comfortable position to receive health care. This could be lying down, sitting down or standing.

- Helping patients on machines and operating tables.

- Choosing the right assistive device for each patient's needs.

- Providing therapy to patients.

Note that ergonomic principles do not benefit patients alone. For example, the right application of procedures for moving patients from one point to another will also prevent injuries and strain on nurses and other health care workers.

Here are a few things nurses should note when handling patients and using common hospital equipment and facilities:

- Do a bit of stretching or warming up before lifting a client or heavy objects.

- Take time to review your actions and what the best procedure for execution might be.

- Collaborate with other health care workers or caregivers. Explain what you want to do and how you want to achieve it. Also communicate with patients so they can physically and emotionally prepare themselves for the activity. In some situations, a patient may even be able to participate in the process, bending, shifting and twisting when needed.

- Always face the person or object you are about to move or lift unless you are working in a group and your positioning at the time might not permit you to face the client.

- Keep key body parts like the spine, neck, back and head aligned when lifting. Avoid twisting.

- When lifting, provide a secure base for supporting yourself by keeping your feet apart.

- Keep a secure grip on the object or client you will lift from the beginning.

- Use the muscles of your arms and legs to lift and not your back.

- Use mechanical lifts and appropriate assistive devices when available.

### *Assess Clients' Ability to Balance, Transfer and Use Assistive Device Prior to Planning Care*

Before assistive devices like crutches, walkers, braces, hearing and visual aids are assigned to patients, they must be tested for client suitability and convenience. Factors like cognitive ability and muscular strength could impact a person's ability to balance and use some devices.

Therefore, every assistive device assigned to a patient must meet individual needs, such as developmental stage, height, weight and terrain. Each patient must also be properly informed on how to use and manage their assistive devices.

### *Provide Instruction and information to Clients about Body Positions that Eliminate the Potential for Repetitive Stress Injuries*

Repetitive stress injuries occur due to repeated movement or overuse of certain muscles or muscle groups. They typically occur due to the postures patients maintain over time or due to placing weight or applying pressure on certain parts of the body over time. Repetitive stress injuries cause cramping, stiffness and neurological discomfort and might lead to complications when not properly attended to.

Patients should be taught to maintain anatomically correct positions and should be made aware of their new limits or restrictions, if any.

### Handling Hazardous and Infectious Materials

Hazardous materials are non-biological materials that pose some form of harm to human beings, animals and other living components of the environment. They can be anything ranging from harmful chemicals and radiation to soiled and used equipment like needles that could become potential sources of infection.

RNs are instrumental in ensuring that these materials, in all their forms, do not pose any risk to clients.

### Identify Biohazardous, Flammable and Infectious Materials

The US Occupational Safety and Health Administration (OSHA) requires that workers in health care environments have firsthand information about hazardous materials, what risks they may pose and what actions to take in the case of exposure. Nurses and other health care workers must also be able to identify these hazardous materials and how to handle them.

Biohazardous materials are biological waste and items that have been contaminated with biological waste that can be harmful to humans. Used hospital bedding, tubes containing bodily fluids and excretions, and used needles are all examples of biohazardous waste.

Biohazardous, flammable, explosive and infectious materials are always regulated at national, state and local levels. Health care facilities should comply with the policies available to their region for labeling, storing, disposing and managing these wastes.

All hazardous materials should be properly labeled such that even lay personnel are able to identify risks. There should be specific labeling that provides information for identifying the nature of each hazardous material.

### Follow Procedures for Handling Biohazardous and Hazardous Materials

Each biohazardous material comes with unique procedures for handling, transportation, disposal and disinfecting, if applicable. Some waste needs to be destroyed as soon as it is used. Other waste can be disinfected before final disposal, while still other waste can be disposed of in containers and made ready for safe reuse. It is, therefore, important that nurses follow the right protocols and procedures for handling waste.

There are general principles for handling biohazardous waste that apply In all health care systems. Some of these include:

- Rigorous handwashing after handling any biohazardous material.

- Proper allocation of trash cans in patient rooms and at strategic points in the health care facility for easy waste disposal.

- Avoid reusing materials such as needles and latex gloves designed for single use.

- Proper cleaning and disinfection of non-single-use materials like certain PPE that comes in contact with biological waste.

- Proper disposal of biohazardous material in accordance with stipulated national, state and local laws.

- Design the right procedures to ensure proper disposal of each kind of waste.

- Ensure safe transportation and proper labeling of hazardous, radiative and flammable substances, such as oxygen and helium tanks.

- Educate clients and their caregivers on handling and disposing of biohazardous waste such as used bedding and bodily fluids.

### Demonstrate Safe Handling Techniques to Staff and Clients

The RN may be obligated to demonstrate how to safely handle hazardous substances to other staff members in the health care environment, as well as clients who are receiving health care. In such situations, the nurse assumes the role of an educator, assessing the learning needs of concerned parties and demonstrating appropriate techniques for handling hazardous materials.

### Ensure Safe Implementation of Internal Radiation Therapy

Long exposure to radiation poses dangerous health risks. Nurses work with X-ray technicians and other professionals handling radioactive equipment to minimize exposure to radiation.

There are three major ways to ensure safety during radiation therapy: time, distance and shielding. Nurses and technicians should ensure clients have the most minimal exposure to radiation by minimizing exposure time, ensuring safe distance and using shielding.

It is also important to implement safe interaction of caregivers, family, friends and other patients with clients currently being treated with radiation therapy.

## Home Safety

Health care does not end at the health care facility. Nurses are crucial in ensuring clients have appropriate instructions in order to ensure a safe transition to the home environment.

### Assess the Need for Client Home Modifications

Nurses, alongside other health care staff such as physical therapists, discharge planners and counselors, work together to assess clients' homes, identify safety concerns and offer solutions or modifications.

Factors like lighting, handrails, slip-proof floors, oxygen tanks and emergency exits are crucial to improving the well-being of patients and helping them adjust their lifestyles to the new health conditions they may be managing.

### Apply Knowledge of Client Pathophysiology to Home Safety Interventions

Certain diseases and disorders require that unique provisions be made for clients so they can better manage these situations. Patients with cognitive disabilities might require close monitoring and may be prevented from exposure to materials that could potentially cause harm to them or others around them. Clients with perceptual deficits will also require special aids that will promote their safety, help them handle emergency situations and help them interact with their environment better.

### *Educate Clients on Safety Issues*

Many clients are unaware of what potential risks their daily routines and lifestyles might impose on their health. Nurses must determine each client's level of knowledge about home safety needs and provide adequate education.

Clients may be presented with written instructions or other teaching aids that will serve as a resource they can always return to.

### *Encourage Clients to Use Protective Equipment when Using Devices that Can Cause Injury*

Clients should be enlightened on the right protective equipment to use for each high-risk activity and should be strongly encouraged to always use this equipment. Protective equipment applicable for home use includes simple items such as hand gloves and safety goggles. Clients should also be encouraged to properly dispose of sharps and other biohazardous wastes.

### *Evaluate Client Care Environment for Fire and Environmental Hazards*

Patient care environments must be properly evaluated for fire and other environmental hazards. Such hazards must be eliminated when possible, while other needed health care materials must be correctly labeled to inform health care personnel of their nature. Lastly, fire safety equipment must always be available and within reach.

### Reporting of Incident/Event/Irregular Occurrence/Violence

Nurses must always report irregular occurrences, cases of violence and other uncommon events, depending on the applicable protocol at their workplace. Usually, such reports must go to the supervising or charge nurse and the risk management department in the health care facility.

Providing these reports helps to ensure issues are promptly addressed and can be prevented in the future. They also help with record-keeping and tracking trends.

Details that should be included in formal reports for incidents and other irregular occurrences include:

- The date, time and place where the event occurred

- A brief background on what triggered the event, such as an object that a client tripped on, for example

- The name of the individual affected by the event

- The nature of injuries sustained

- The names of the witnesses present

- The care and treatment procedures that were used

- The names of health care workers who were contacted to attend to the event

*Identify Needs/Situations where Reporting of Incident/Event/Irregular Occurrence is Appropriate*

Only events that are truly abnormal should be recorded. These include:

**Practitioner Variance:** This is an irregular occurrence that is a consequence of the activities or services provided by a health care provider. An example includes delayed attendance to a client until complications occur.

**System or Institutional Violence:** This is an irregular occurrence that is associated with some excesses on the part of the health care facility. A popular example is occurrences due to inadequacy of supplies or shortage of staff members.

**Patient Variance:** This is an irregular occurrence associated with excesses on the part of the client. For example, unexplainable and sudden complications or an event that occurs because a client has not adhered to a treatment routine.

### Acknowledge and Document Practice Errors and Near Misses

RNs, as well as other health care providers, must remain responsible at all times and own up to human errors in the workplace. These errors, when identified, should be properly documented with details on the exact nature of the error, the consequences that accompanied it and the current state of those affected by such errors.

Errors and near-misses remain under-reported in health care facilities. This is due to various factors, such as fear of owning up and getting penalized, ignorance of the error itself and ignorance of how to go about documenting such errors. Proper documentation can, however, help inform intervention procedures, including how health care workers should be trained to reduce the frequency of such errors occurring in the future.

### Evaluate Response to Error/Event/Occurrence

The RN must immediately evaluate a client's response to an error or negative occurrence as soon as such an event has been identified. Most times, clients are not able to provide information on the effects of such occurrences as they may be unconscious, unaware of their situation or too indisposed to communicate.

The nurse should perform a thorough evaluation to identify the patient's current state while paying attention to priority needs first. The patient's state at the time of occurrence should be recorded and progress should be tracked over time.

### Report, Intervene and/or Escalate Unsafe Practices of Health Care Personnel

RNs are responsible for looking out for other health care workers and reporting out-of-place behaviors and unsafe practices that could pose threats to clients and other persons in the health care environment. Such unsafe practices include substance abuse, improper care, biases directed toward certain clients, degenerating health and mental state of a health worker and so on.

## Safe Use of Equipment

The state of equipment used in the health care environment and how staff members are able to manage such equipment go a long way toward preventing hazards, client complications and injuries to health care workers.

### *Inspect Equipment for Safety Hazards*

All equipment used, whether by staff members or clients, should be inspected for what potential risks it may pose to users and those around the equipment. Thorough equipment inspection and evaluation are usually conducted by the maintenance or equipment department. Nurses can ensure that these inspection procedures have been observed and should pay attention to instructions and operation procedures, including preliminary checks that are necessary before using any equipment.

Nurses should particularly look out for frayed electrical cords, overloaded power outlets, loose or missing equipment parts and other questionable conditions that could pose a threat.

### *Teach Clients about the Safe Use of Health Care Equipment*

Both clients and staff members should be properly trained to handle and manage whatever equipment they may be using. They should also learn how to identify potential threats and handle quick fixes if applicable, as well as what to do in the face of complications.

Clients should be trained on how to safely handle equipment, particularly any they will use at home, away from staff members' oversight. This equipment should be thoroughly checked before being provided to clients, and clients should be taught how to make personal routine checks. Depending on the nature of the equipment or device, they may also be instructed to bring it for inspection or replacement during their next health check.

## Facilitate Appropriate and Safe Use of Equipment

RNs can help facilitate the appropriate and safe use of equipment by doing the following:

- Learning how each piece of equipment works.

- Ensuring they do not operate any equipment unless they have been trained to handle it.

- Performing routine inspections on equipment before use and reporting malfunctions as soon as they are discovered.

- Not using equipment or devices deemed faulty.

- Educating other staff members about how to handle equipment when they are in the capacity to do so.

- Educating clients on how to properly manage equipment and assistive devices.

- Reporting equipment that is faulty or out of use so it can be labeled accordingly or removed to prevent another staff member from using it.

## Remove Malfunctioning Equipment from the Client Care Area and Report the Problem to the Appropriate Personnel

Faulty equipment should not be disposed of unless it has been designated irreparable by a professional technician. That said, faulty equipment should be removed to a place where it can be properly checked and fixed.

## Security Plans

Security planning is an important aspect of health care. An excellent security plan ensures lives and properties at the facility are always secured from safety concerns such as newborn theft, stealing of clients' and family members' belongings and even major security concerns such as bomb threats.

## Use Clinical Decision-Making/Critical Thinking in Situations Related to Security Planning

Once again, critical thinking and excellent decision-making skills are crucial in security planning. The RN is a key participant in the planning, execution and evaluation of security procedures and must be able to offer working solutions at all times.

In accordance with regulations and recommendations by security bodies, health care facilities must create working security plans. Bodies responsible for providing security regulations include the JCAHO, the International Association for Health Care Security and Safety and The Centers for Medicare and Medicaid.

Nurses must remain fully aware and updated about the security plans in their facility, including codes for communicating situations and what to do in the event of a security threat.

## Apply Principles of Triage and Evacuation Procedures and Protocols

In the event of a security threat, the nurse must apply principles of triage to create a protocol that caters to the most critical clients first. These include immobile clients who may be unable to escape threats on their own or those who have been critically injured due to such threats. As explained in the principles of triage, medically unstable patients are to be attended to first, followed by stable patients who still require assistance and lastly, ambulatory clients who do not require assistance.

## Follow Security Plan and Procedures

Security threats are a unique form of emergency, and nurses must always be prepared to combat them. Key ways to do this are periodic training, reviewing policies, procedures and recommendations for different security situations and participating in mock sessions to prepare for situations like access breaches, violence and property or human theft.

## Standard Precautions/Transmission-Based Precautions/Surgical Asepsis

Infection control is just as crucial as other safety measures. Because the health care environment is one where patients and health care providers interact with several potential infection risk factors all at once, it is highly important to ensure that infections are not transmitted from one patient to the other, between health care personnel or from patients to health care personnel and vice versa.

There are several procedures for infection control, such as maintaining a strict surgical asepsis routine, properly disposing of biohazardous waste and following standard and transmission-based precautionary measures.

### Understand Communicable Diseases and the Modes of Organism Transmission

Diseases are transmitted when an etiologic agent, that is, a pathogen capable of causing an infection, is transmitted from a current host or reservoir to a new or susceptible host. Disease-causing agents include bacteria, fungi, viruses and helminth parasites. These agents go through a chain of transmission from the reservoir to the portal of exit, to the mode of transmission to the portal of entry and finally to the susceptible host. This is known as the chain of infection.

The portal of exit is the point through which the agent or pathogen leaves the reservoir, while the portal of entry is the point through which the agent enters a susceptible host. These portals can include body orifices or systems and activities like sneezing or vomiting.

When pathogens leave through the portal of exit of a reservoir, they may gain access to the portal of entry of a new host, like another patient, a medical staff member or family, friends and well-wishers of patients.

The mode of transmission is the specific medium through which the infectious agent is transmitted from the reservoir to a new host. Modes of transmission of pathogens are:

- Contact (direct and indirect)

- Airborne

- Droplet

- Vector-borne

### Assess Client Care Area for Sources of Infection

RNs must continually monitor and assess the client care area for potential sources of infection while providing health care to patients. Infection sources and risk factors for infections should be properly communicated and the right measures for preventing, testing for or treating such infections should be taken immediately.

Because nurses and other staff members are important figures in transmitting health care-acquired infections, they must strictly follow preventive procedures, including frequent handwashing and use of PPE.

### Apply Principles of Infection Prevention

There are several provisions for infection prevention and control that nurses must strictly adhere to at all times. These include:

**Hand hygiene:** Hand hygiene is the most effective procedure for preventing the spread of infection. Proper hand hygiene, such as washing with mild soap and water, disinfecting when necessary and wearing protective gloves, prevents thousands of infections from spreading in health care environments. Nurses should note that, unlike medical equipment that can be sterilized, the hands and other parts of the skin cannot be sterilized. They can only be sanitized. Sterilization procedures such as the use of bleach and other chemicals are harmful to the skin and could cause irritation or more serious skin concerns.

Handwashing should be done:

- Before and after contact with a client

- Before and after removing gloves

- After touching equipment, instruments and other treatment materials with bare hands

- When hands have been soiled with bodily fluids, secretions and chemicals

**Aseptic Techniques:** Aseptic techniques or medical asepsis are measures taken in addition to standard and transmission-based precautions to prevent the transfer of disease-causing organisms from one person or object to the other. Aseptic techniques include barriers, patient and equipment preparation, environmental controls and contact guidelines. They differ from sterile techniques, which are measures for neutralizing infectious microorganisms. Sterile techniques are usually applied during surgical procedures and invasive wound care.

**Universal/Standard Precautions:** These are recognized infection control measures for preventing infection spread among clients, whether or not they've been diagnosed with any infection.

**Transmission-Based Precautions:** These are preventive and infection control measures that are utilized to combat and inhibit the spread of specific infections. These precautionary procedures are informed based on the type of infection and its medium of transmission.

**PPE:** This is specialized equipment used to protect specific body areas from injury and exposure to infectious agents. Examples of PPEs are gloves, goggles, masks, respirators, aprons, face shields and gowns. Nurses should observe basic principles for donning, removing, disposing of and sterilizing personal PPE as appropriate. They should also wash their hands before and after using PPE.

### Follow Correct Policies and Procedures when Reporting a Client with a Communicable Disease

Infectious diseases can spread very quickly and become a major threat to the whole community. Nurses should follow the regulations that apply to reporting and communicating diseases. Usually, reports about communicable diseases, epidemics and other outbreaks are submitted to the Centers for Disease Control and Prevention.

### Educate Client and Staff Regarding Infection Prevention Measures

RNs directly and indirectly educate clients and staff members on infection prevention and control measures. They assess the educational needs of these groups and plan educational activities to meet those needs. They also evaluate the impact and effectiveness of such educational sessions on infection prevention and control.

Nurses may educate clients on infection prevention measures based on their specific health needs, current health care routine and life situation. They teach clients how to properly dispose of biohazardous waste, how to perform asepsis and other standard or treatment-based precautions.

Nurses are responsible for helping patients and their family members understand the importance of certain infection control and prevention measures, such as isolation and the need for family members to wear a gown or other PPE before accessing treatment wards.

### Use Appropriate Precautions for Immunocompromised Clients

Immunocompromised clients are at a higher risk of contracting infection after exposure. This state may also be worsened by other risk factors such as an immune-deficiency disease, age, medications and certain therapeutic interventions like radiation and chemotherapy.

Immunocompromised clients are given special care and prevented from contact with infectious agents that might not pose a threat to non-compromised clients. Stringent infection control measures should be practiced for these clients. They may need to be isolated from other people until they have attained some level of recovery and immunity.

*Use Appropriate Technique to Set up a Sterile Field/Maintain Asepsis*

Nurses may assist or manage the process of setting up a sterile field during surgical asepsis. Here are the appropriate techniques and procedures to follow:

- Only sterile items should be placed on the sterile field.

- The nurse should never have the sterile field below the waist level.

- The nurse should not lean over or turn their back to the sterile field.

- Coughing or sneezing over the sterile field contaminates it.

- There should be a one-inch border of sterile space around the sterile field. It is within this space that sterile items are placed.

- Moisture or wetness contaminates the sterile field. It must remain dry at all times.

- Sterile liquids should be carefully poured into sterile containers on the sterile field while ensuring the liquid does not run over or cover the label of bottles and other containers.

- All staff around a sterile field should wear gowns and gloves. Those working directly on the sterile field should use sterile masks.

### Evaluate Infection Control Precautions Implemented by Staff Members

Nurses directly and indirectly watch out for themselves and other staff members to ensure they adhere to the right infection control and prevention measures. They can offer immediate education to staff who have not properly learned the various infection prevention procedures and can be involved in planning, designing and evaluating the results of more organized educational activities for staff members.

### Evaluate Whether Aseptic Technique is Performed Correctly

Aseptic techniques should be carried out in accordance with generally accepted procedures. Nurses should evaluate and monitor the process to ascertain staff members' competency and that they have correctly adhered to the procedures.

### Use of Restraints/Safety Devices

Restraints and other safety devices may be required in situations where mobility can increase the risk of falls or where there is a risk of suicide or self-harm.

### Assess the Appropriateness of the Type of Restraint/Safety Device Used

There are different kinds of restraints that can be used depending on the situation. They include:

- Using belts, jackets and other devices that will prevent limb movement.

- Holding down a patient in order to restrict movement.

- Isolating the patient in one room without providing a means of exit.

- Using medicines that will keep the patient immobile for a prescribed time.

### Follow Requirements when Using Restraints

Ethical considerations and individual restraint requirements must be kept in mind. Heavy restraints should only be used as a last resort when other control measures are ineffective. Restraints should not be used as punishment, and restraining measures should not cause further harm to the patient.

Nurses should be trained on how to use restraints appropriately.

Patient rights and ethics must also be considered when using restraints. National and state laws on the use of restraints must be followed, and the concerns of family members of patients who are being restrained must also be acknowledged.

Patients who are under restraints must be put on special care, as they will need help moving their bowels, eating and being kept clean. Restrained patients should not remain in the same position for long to prevent cramps and bed sores. Patients who can speak and are conscious of their environment should be allowed to communicate their inconveniences so they can be properly cared for.

Lastly, all restraining procedures should be properly documented.

### Monitor/Evaluate Client Response to Restraints/Safety Devices

Patients who are under restraints should be closely monitored to prevent further harm. A restraint should be removed immediately if it poses a threat to the patient. Nurses should look out for signs like difficulty in breathing, pallor, blue skin and choking when restraints are used. Nurses should also periodically check for optimal blood flow and watch out for numbness, peeling and bruises at points where restraints are attached.

Restraints should be removed as soon as patients are healthy and conscious enough not to cause harm to themselves and others.

# Chapter 2: Health Promotion and Maintenance

## Aging Process

Aging comes with challenges, and people respond to these challenges differently. It is, therefore, important for a nurse to identify and assess the responses of individuals to these changes and challenges as they occur.

For some infants, the changes associated with weaning might produce a defiant reaction. Others might have difficulties adapting to toilet training or the arrival of a younger sibling. School-aged children might have challenges adapting to school routines, and older kids might react to puberty differently.

For young adults, there are usually significant changes associated with higher responsibilities like marriage, pregnancy and childbirth. Some adults might adapt positive coping mechanisms, cherishing the journey and experience. In contrast, others might adopt maladaptive coping mechanisms, resulting in total disgust for the body changes and accompanying responsibilities.

Older adults must adapt to changes in their bodies as they get slower and become unable to perform all the activities they once used to at the same pace. This stage can also be filled with the possibility of regrets over decisions that should or should not have been made. There is a feeling of loneliness and isolation at this stage.

Irrespective of the stage of life that clients are in, it is the responsibility of a trained nurse to quickly assess clients' reactions to these changes.

The nurse should note patients that are adapting or have adapted well and those who have maladaptive reactions.

# Provide care and education for newborns, infants and toddlers from birth through 2 years of age

## Neonates

The World Health Organization (WHO) defines neonates as children newly born up to 28 days of age. At this stage, children have the highest chances of developing complications which can result in death. Hence, it is the duty of the nurse to be vigilant for any signs of ill health in the neonate.

Since neonates cannot speak or complain, the observation skills of the nurse must be top-notch. At birth, the first assessment is the APGAR score. This is a fast way of evaluating the status of a child at birth. APGAR stands for Appearance, Pulse, Grimace, Activity and Respiration.

- Appearance: The nurse should examine if the neonate is pink all around, has a pink body with bluish extremities or is bluish all around.
- Pulse: The pulse should be checked to see if it is absent, less than 100 beats per minute or greater than 100 beats per minute.
- Grimace: A neonate should be assessed for if a grimace is absent, minimal or responds to a prompt to stimulation.
- Activity: Activity can either be absent, weak flexion of the arms and legs or the neonate crying and actively moving body parts.
- Respiration: Respiration is evaluated as either absent, slow, irregular or good, with vigorous crying.

Each parameter in the APGAR score is assessed as either 0, 1 or 2 and the total is added up to 10. If a child is less than 4, then the child is in severe distress and needs urgent intensive care and resuscitation. Four to 6 is moderately distressed and requires moderate attention and resuscitation. Neonates scored 7 and above are in excellent condition.

Gestational age is another parameter that is used to assess a neonate. To measure the gestational age, the New Ballard Scale is used. This scale is based on both physical maturity and the maturity of the neuromuscular system. It is graded from -1 to 5 and measures the following parameters:

- Posture, square window, which refers to the movement of the wrist (varies from greater than 90 degrees to 0 degrees)
- Arm recoil (ranges from 180 degrees to less than 90 degrees)
  Scarf sign (neonate crossing arms over chest)
- Heel-to-ear movement.

The normal size of a neonate ranges from a length of 18 to 22 inches and 12.5 to 14.5 inches due to the head circumference, and the normal weight is from 5 pounds, 8 ounces to 8 pounds, 13 ounces.

- Vital signs: Respiratory rate 30 to 60 breaths per minute.
- Pulse: 100 to 140 bpm.
- Blood pressure: 60/40 to 80/50 mmHg.
- Temperature: 97.7 to 98.9 degrees Fahrenheit.

Abdomen: Full, round, moves with respiration, bowel sounds present within a few hours of birth, umbilical site clean and free of discharge or discoloration.

Head: Head circumference within normal range, eyes bilaterally equal in size and shape. Observe eye movements. Ears should be placed at normal levels bilaterally; low-set ears and abnormal position of eyes and nose can be suggestive of Down syndrome.

The mouth should have a closed oral palate, with pi oral mucosa and bilaterally symmetrical lip and tongue movements. Observe for excessive salivation, which might be a sign of a tracheoesophageal fistula.

Neonate skin should be pink without sustained blueness, jaundice or cyanosis. Lanugo hair, vernix caseosa and telangiectatic nevi might also be present.

Fontanels should be soft and fat, with no depression or bulge. Bulging can be a sign of raised intracranial depression, while depression can be a sign of reduced intracranial pressure, which can be due to dehydration. Molding might be present if the delivery was vaginal.

Excretory and urogenital systems: Meconium should be passed within a day of birth. Male testes should be properly descended in the testicles; presence of the prepuce over the glans and rugae in the scrotum. Some females may have some level of swelling in the labia and blood from the vagina.

**Infants**

Infants are greater than 28 days and up to one year of age. At this age, infants are in Erikson's first stage of development, the trust vs. mistrust stage. At this stage, infants expect everything they need in terms of food, love, care, warmth and security to be provided by their caregivers. If these needs are unmet, the child can develop a feeling of mistrust and that adults are not dependable.

This stage also coincides with Piaget's first phase of cognitive development in children, known as the sensorimotor stage. At this stage, children learn about their surroundings through their sensory and motor activities.

**What to expect**

- Suckle reflex
- Grasping reflex
- Moving eyes and focusing on objects for limited periods
- Cooing and babbling
- Responding to sudden movement or loud noises and some selected words
- Doubled birth weight by the first birthday
- Teeth begin to develop
- Increase in length (1 inch per month until 1 year)
- Increase in head circumference

- Ability to transfer objects from hand to hand (usually at about 9 months)
- The child forms bonds with parents and caregivers
- Separation anxiety sets in at this stage
- Feeding every two hours with formula or breast milk. (The WHO recommends exclusive breastfeeding for babies in the first six months of life.)

## Toddler (1–3 years of age)

Some call this developmental stage the terrible twos because children begin to explore and exhibit some defiant behavior and tantrums.

Children at this age are now at Erikson's second stage of development, which is known as autonomy vs. shame and doubt. At this stage, children are focused on the development of self-control. They usually want to push the boundaries of the things they can do on their own or require help to do. At this stage, they do things impulsively, act out of curiosity and they become very energetic.

They might not like the rules that are set in place, as they want to do things on their terms. This might lead to frustration, tantrums and inappropriate behavior.

At this stage they should learn and master potty training.

Parents and caregivers are expected to provide opportunities for the toddler to make some independent decisions, no matter how small. This might be anything from selecting snacks to eat to what clothes to wear.

## Provide care and education for preschool, school-age and adolescent clients ages 3 through 17 years

### Preschoolers (3–5 years)

This stage coincides with Erikson's third stage of psychosocial development. It is called the initiative vs. guilt stage. Here, the child begins to exert some level of dominance and control over the world around him.

The initiative part of this stage allows children to try out new activities and explore experiences in play. Children begin to explore the power of imagination and the freedom to create.

Failure to successfully complete a task or overcome an obstacle can lead to a feeling of shame and guilt in children at this stage. It is a "good" versus "bad" situation for children. They are "good" if they excel in tasks and "bad" if they do not.

At this stage, children are refining motor skills. This is the stage at which disabilities affecting development are more obvious. They typically experience a weight gain of about four to seven pounds in a year and then increase about two to three inches in height.

**What to expect**

- Able to stand on one foot for longer than 10 seconds
- Able to hop around
- Draw a person with features
- Follow simple and clear directions
- Decrease in separation anxiety
- Able to express feelings and desires verbally
- Dress and undress on their own
- Need reassurance and encouragement to always try again if they fail at any tasks
- Failure should not be why they do not attempt new tasks or experiences
- Children at this stage should be allowed to take the initiative in play or explore their surroundings as long as it does not put them or others in danger

**The School-Aged Child (6–12 years)**

At this stage, the child is now at what Erikson termed the industry vs. inferiority stage. Here, the child begins to learn about accomplishments and abilities. At this stage, the child begins to associate success with competence and a feeling of superiority, while failure is met with feelings of inferiority. If children at this stage are always encouraged and praised, they will develop a corresponding sense of competence and belief in themselves.

Piaget's cognitive development theory places children at this age in the concrete operational stage. Here, they are able to solve problems by considering several angles, outcomes and perspectives. They can also solve problems that have to do with conservation. Conservation is an ideology of seeing that things are the same, even if they look different. Solving problems related to conservation is useful in solving mathematical problems and word problems, which are key skills required of this age group.

**What to expect**

- Challenge authority figures around them
- Follow complicated commands
- Perform actions that require combining several motions
- Retain information
- Prefer same-gender friends and peers
- Emulate their parents of the same sex
- Recall names, addresses, ages, best food and personal details
- Menarche might develop, as well as other secondary sexual characteristics

**Adolescents**

The WHO defines this age group as 10 to 19 years old.

Erikson defines it as the identity vs. confusion stage. Here, teenagers develop a sense of identity. This sense of identity goes a long way in determining the type of people that they will be in life. If this identity is well determined, the individual will usually be stable. If the teenager is unable to do so, they might become confused and develop a weak sense of identity and self.

Piaget describes this as the formal operational stage, where there is a lot of abstract thinking. Teenagers can think about abstract concepts easily, even those that are not rational or realistic. They can also apply reasoning skills to solve problems in a more coordinated and systematic manner.

At this stage, they share normal vital signs with adults. There is an increased need for calories due to the growth spurt that takes place in this stage. Completion of sexual maturity occurs in this stage.

**What to expect**

- Attraction toward the opposite sex
- Self-conscious
- Seek peer group acceptance

## Provide care and education for adult clients ages 18 through 64 years

**Young Adults**

Young adults between 19 and 35 are at the intimacy vs. isolation stage, according to Erikson. Here, they begin to form closer, stronger relationships with other people.

**What to expect**

- Seeking purpose in life
- Healthy coping mechanisms develop to deal with the demands of work, relationships and other commitments
- Preventive steps are taken to reduce the occurrence of chronic conditions as they age

**Middle age**

This typically begins after the age of 40 and lasts until the age of 60. Muscular strength begins to decline. There is a reduction in sexual drive, and menopause and erectile dysfunction may occur at this stage.

Individuals in this stage are at what Erikson termed the generativity vs. stagnation stage. Adults at this stage are concerned with a need to produce structures, people and things that will outlive them. They are also very concerned about impacting the world and improving the lives of others.

**What to expect**

- Worries ranging from the care of children to the care of aging parents
- Diagnoses of chronic health conditions
- Concerned with structures that outlive them

## Provide care and education for adult client ages 65 years and over

This is the final stage of psychosocial development and it is seen in the elderly. It is called the integrity vs. despair stage, and people at this point usually look in retrospect at the influence of the choices they made earlier in life. They either sit back to regret the effect of their decisions, leading to despair, or are happy with the outcomes they see regarding the meaning and purpose of their lives.

**What to expect:**

- Gradual decline in physical function and musculature
- Sensorineural changes: Decreased ability to see, hear, smell and touch, slower reaction times and night blindness
- Cardiovascular system: Reduced cardiac output, stroke volume, reduced venous return
- Musculoskeletal: Decrease in muscle mass, muscle tone and strength, degenerating joints, bones and reductions in intervertebral disc spaces
- Renal changes: Reduction of kidney size, decreased creatinine clearance and glomerular function
- Hepatic changes result in reduced hepatic blood flow and metabolism, leading to reduced hepatic clearance and a subsequent increase in the concentrations of medications in the body.

- Skin changes: Wrinkling, increased skin fragility, graying of hair, dry skin, reduced turgor and elasticity, thicker nails
- Respiratory system: Reduced lung expansion, increased risk of respiratory infections
- Fluid and electrolyte changes.
- Reminiscing over accomplishments or regrets in life
- Increase in the occurrence of sickness and death
- Retirement.
- Need to change the environment to adapt to needs
- Require more assistance in performing daily activities

Great care should be taken when medication is prescribed for older adults. There is a significant impairment in drug distribution, absorption and clearance in this age group, and the nurse must be very conscious of this when attending to older individuals.

## Pre-/Intra-/Postpartum and Newborn Care

### Assess the client's psychosocial response to pregnancy

The period of pregnancy places emotional demands on anyone, both the mother and father of the child as well as relatives. There are varying levels of psychological reactions when a pregnancy is announced, whether it is expected or not.

Some concerns around pregnancy can include fear of body changes, financial burdens, anxiety, concerns over delivery, the safety of the fetus and more.

Some people have strong family support that helps them through pregnancy, while others do not.

### Assess the client for symptoms of postpartum complications

After childbirth, there is a risk of postpartum complications, especially hemorrhage if delivery was via SVD. Postpartum hemorrhage can be prevented by active management of the third stage of labor. This involves administering 10 IU of oxytocin per minute after delivery to help the uterus contract, ensuring that the entire placenta is delivered through controlled cord traction, and uterine massage.

The nurse checks for malfunctions in reproductive organs, records and reports any abnormal changes and provides nursing interventions as fast as possible. Examination of vital signs, weight, amount of blood loss, intake and output, mental state, etc., is also important.

Assessment for the risk of vaginal, uterine or cervical infections after childbirth is done by looking out for symptoms of fever, itching, swelling, redness and other presenting signs.

## Calculate the expected delivery date

A pregnant mother is expected to know the date to anticipate when she will have her baby. This is relayed during prenatal clinics, and the nursing officer can educate mothers on how to estimate dates between 36 and 40 weeks of pregnancy.

For example, a woman who is pregnant can run ultrasound scans to determine EDDs but can also manually calculate dates using the last menstrual cycle date preceding the pregnancy.

## Check fetal heart rate during routine prenatal exams

At the clinic, pregnant mothers are usually educated by nursing officers on the importance of prenatal care, including listening to the fetal heart rate, which is examined by ultrasound.

The nurse can check for signs of distress in pregnancy resulting from an increased fetal heart rate of up to 200 BPM, which is often associated with uterine conditions or maternal health issues such as hypertension, infections, sepsis, certain lifestyles and medication.

## Assist client with learning and performing newborn care

The nurse is responsible for educating new mothers on how to care for their newborns. This includes breastfeeding newborns, bathing, caring for the umbilical cord, diapering and cleaning and caring for the baby's feeding items if the child is not breastfed.

Also, the nurse teaches mothers how to monitor the growth and development of their children according to the developmental milestones chart.

## Provide prenatal care and education

Prenatal care involves health education and assessment for pregnancy risks or unhealthy behaviors of mothers, such as smoking, drinking alcohol, stress and so on.

Pregnant women are counseled during prenatal clinics about the importance of practicing health-compliant behaviors, especially the impact on the unborn baby's cognitive and mental state.

Diagnostic tests, blood tests to check for infections (HIV, Hepatitis B), blood sugar levels, rhesus factors, vital signs monitoring and weight assessments are all done in prenatal care to prevent or reduce the risk of adverse events during labor.

During prenatal care and education, a mother will also be taught about nutritional needs, such as meals or supplements essential for the baby, the need for regular clinic visits, childbirth methods and how to deal with multiple gestation.

## Provide care and education to a prepartum client or a client in labor

In the four stages of labor, the client is expected to be aware of presenting symptoms. The nurse is also expected to be ready for complications that can arise at any of these stages. This is highlighted to the pregnant mother with coping techniques to adopt for the safe delivery of the baby.

Nursing interventions are key at this point. The nurse provides emergency care and seeks the safety of the client. Patient exercise, hygiene, dilation checks against labor and fetal heartbeat are monitored. Several delivery methods are presented to the client as appropriate. These include vaginal delivery, cesarean section, forceps delivery and water birth.

The consequences or complications of whatever method is chosen should also be communicated to the client, especially when there is a breech position, preeclampsia symptoms, tachycardia or other cardiac abnormalities. The relatives are educated on the importance of caring for the client and providing all necessary support.

## Provide postpartum care and education

Before discharge, postpartum care is given to the mother, which will enable her to handle her health and that of the newborn. The nurse is charged with the duty of examining the client and providing adequate information about hygiene, childcare, feeding and complications such as hemorrhage and sepsis.

Education on the care of the reproductive organs, use of analgesics, mother and child attachment, laboratory scans and family planning methods are given to women who opt for vaginal delivery.

The client is informed on how to reach out to health care practitioners for further review, especially when symptoms of postpartum psychosis are suspected.

## Provide discharge instructions (postpartum and newborn care)

Before a newborn is discharged, the mother is instructed on how to handle emergencies and look out for noticeable changes in hair, skin color and so on.

Also, education is provided on how to bathe the newborn, prevent exposure to cold, wash hands before handling clothing and feeding items, as well as the nutritional benefits of breastfeeding.

In the case of a young woman who has just had a baby and is expected to meet the demands of a paid job after a few weeks, the nurse can advise against possible stress.

## Evaluate the client's ability to care for the newborn

The client is expected to demonstrate all procedures, and the nurse verifies an understanding of the client's ability to independently care for the newborn.

Observation sessions can be conducted, or role-play trials can be used to see that the client understands the necessities of newborn care, such as cleaning the umbilical cord, medication administration, circumcision, breastfeeding, bottle feeding, putting a baby to sleep, comfortable carrying of the newborn, perineal care and more.

# Health Screening

Health screening is an essential part of health promotion and maintenance.

## Apply knowledge of pathophysiology to health screening

To effectively perform health screening, nurses must be able to apply knowledge of the disease process or progression. They must be able to identify the signs and symptoms of disease progression to detect or diagnose a condition as fast as possible. When an express diagnosis is impossible, they can refer clients for further investigations.

Examples of routine screening examinations which should be performed in different populations include:

- Blood sugar: Blood sugar can be checked while fasting (known as fasting blood sugar) and not fasting (known as random blood sugar). A fasting patient should typically not have a blood sugar that exceeds 100 mg/dL, but some researchers allow a reading up to 125 mg/dl, while a patient's random blood sugar should not exceed 199 mg/dl. If any of these values are out of range, it indicates a need for further testing. An understanding of the pathophysiology of diabetes mellitus, which could cause a rise in blood sugar, informs this screening. If the condition is in a younger adult, it is more likely to be Type I, and if it is in an elderly patient, it is more likely to be Type II. Further tests are required to confirm the diagnosis, such as HBA1C or FLP.

- Blood pressure check: A routine screening checks the systolic and diastolic blood pressure. The expected normal blood pressure is 120/80 mmHg. An understanding of the pathophysiology of hypertension, which raises blood pressure, informs this screening. Hypertension is technically defined as blood pressure greater than 140/90 mmHg. However, there are stages of pre-hypertension that occur before crossing 140/90 mmHg, followed by stage I and stage II.

Diagnosis is made after at least two readings taken at separate times are persistently above the normal values.

- A fasting lipid profile is a test used to diagnose high cholesterol levels. Adults should do this test at least once every five years. It detects the levels of total cholesterol.

- Colorectal screening: For adults over 50 years of age, colorectal screening should be done regularly. Knowledge of the pathophysiology of colorectal cancer informs this screening in this age group since it is most common in them. The screening might include colonoscopy, sigmoidoscopy, digital rectal examination, fecal occult and blood testing.

- Breast cancer screening: This is very important in all women of 40 years and above. A mammogram should be done at earlier ages for women who have a family or personal history of breast cancer or a breast pathology such as a mass or lump. Several health awareness campaigns advocate for breast self-examination among women.

**Perform health history/health and risk assessments**

A health history is one of the most significant ways of obtaining health information from clients.

A nurse must be aware of the two classifications of data:

- Primary data and secondary data: Primary data refers to data that is collected directly from the client or patient. Here, you receive the information directly. Primary data also includes data that a nurse obtains from observation or examination of the client. Secondary data is obtained from other sources, such as relatives, medical records and other health care personnel.

- Objective and subjective data: Objective data refers to data that can be measured and observed objectively. It can be seen, felt or touched and the inferences made from it are largely unquestionable. Subjective data, however, cannot be objectively measured. It is based on the feelings and biases of either the health care personnel or the client and is usually subject to change. A very good example is pain measurement in which a patient might describe a grade of 8/10. Another patient with more resilience and a higher pain threshold could describe pain as a 5/10.

Taking a detailed health history is done in an interview style. This interview can be carried out with both open and closed-ended questions. Open-ended questions give clients an opportunity to express themselves and talk freely about their complaints. For instance, "What brings you to the emergency department today?" or "What were you doing when you started feeling the headache?"

Close-ended questions are suitable for "Yes" or "No" types of questions, such as, "Do you have children?" or "Are you married?"

A health history should include the full biodata, the presenting complaints, the history of presenting complaints and past medical and surgical history, including things like previous admissions and diagnoses, psychological history and family and social history.

## Performing targeted screening assessments

Routine screening is done to detect conditions that are very general to a specific group of people or the general population. However, target screening can be done when some people show strong tendencies, signs or symptoms of a particular condition or disease.

This target screening is also done when a client is at risk of a certain ailment, or there is a need to rule out a possible condition.

For instance, a child who is not gaining the expected weight and not feeding well might need a nutritional assessment. A child having difficulty reading from far distances might need a visual acuity test performed. A student who begins to act withdrawn, with a loss of interest in formerly enjoyed activities, might need an evaluation of mental status. This is not routinely done, but a targeted screening assessment can be done based on the observed symptoms.

**Utilizing the appropriate interviewing techniques when taking the client's history**

It is not just good enough to know how and when to use open and close-ended questions when interviewing clients. Nurses must also know there are other elements of an excellent interview that should be implemented to make it easier to get information from the client.

- Be open, trusting and nonjudgmental: No matter what the condition is, be open to understanding clients' perspectives, even if what they say is not correct from a professional stance. Sometimes listening allows clients to show areas where they need more help.
- Ensure confidentiality at all times: Every patient has a right to privacy, and this includes asking questions and discussing issues that are private to them. Create an atmosphere free of distractions so that the patient feels safe and comfortable enough to speak. This might mean you need to ask relatives to wait or step aside from the patient when you require information.
- Eliminate communication barriers. Language, for instance, might be a barrier and require an interpreter's presence.
- Use excellent communication techniques. Apply all the knowledge of communication that you have gathered over time. Utilize open and close-ended sentences, active listening and more.
- Speak to relatives when needed: Do not hesitate to speak to relatives when they need to be consulted over an issue. Also, when patients are not able to answer

questions about their health and/or they did not leave an advance directive, then the relative should make that call.

- Cross-check all data with the client to avoid errors. Patients should always say their names in full. All data should be clearly and professionally documented.

All these techniques are important and determine how successful the nurse is in getting the required information from the patient.

## Assess client lifestyle practice risks that may impact health

High-risk behaviors are actions that significantly increase the likelihood of client harm, disease or death. Most of these are modifiable behaviors that are based on choice. They can include diet choices, a sedentary lifestyle, violence and drug abuse, among others.

Biologically, some risks are evident based on race, age and gender and cannot be modified. For instance, the female gender has a higher chance of breast cancer than the male gender. In the same vein, prostate cancer is seen in males. Depression is seen more in females, but suicide is more common in males. Some races have a higher propensity to certain ailments than others.

But high-risk behaviors can be modified, either by stopping the activities altogether or replacing them. Nurses must be able to recognize behaviors that significantly impact the lives of their clients. Examples include:

- Excessive exposure to the sun
- Sedentary lifestyle
- Unbalanced diet
- Smoking cigarettes or other tobacco products
- Alcoholism
- Drug abuse
- Engaging in unprotected sexual intercourse
- Lack of sleep or adequate rest

Nurses must be able to assess clients and their lifestyles to recognize high-risk behaviors that can influence their health in the short and long term.

## High-Risk Behaviors

### Assist clients in identifying behaviors/risks that may impact health

Beyond identifying high-risk behaviors, nurses must also be able to help clients to identify the harm these behaviors are causing or can cause to their health. This is done primarily by client education. Clients must be helped to see some of the unsafe practices that they are engaged in. For instance, a man being admitted for a case of hypertension who still engages in serial drinking and smoking must be made to see the effects of his lifestyle choices on his health.

Clients should be counseled appropriately about the effects of their lifestyle choices and how to change them.

### Educate clients about the prevention and treatment of high-risk health behaviors

After pointing out the high-risk behaviors, it's the responsibility of the nurse to share practical steps that can be taken to eliminate them.

A patient who has been having regular unprotected sex can be counseled on abstinence or using condoms to reduce the risk of contracting STIs. Nurses can also counsel patients on the need to use contraception to prevent unwanted or unplanned pregnancies.

For instance, a patient struggling with smoking habits can be referred to a psychologist or therapist for help.

Some age groups have higher risks of death from automobile accidents. Nurses can provide counsel on prevention, such as the use of seat belts, ensuring all vehicles are in good condition before driving and avoiding driving while intoxicated.

The most important thing is that the steps are easy to understand and practical to take.

# Health Promotion/Disease Prevention

Health promotion is one of the core components of nursing care.

## Assess and educate clients about health risks based on family, population and community

There are several health risks that individuals are exposed to daily. Some of these risks are based on the patients' age, socioeconomic status, hobbies, lifestyle choices, location and population.

Individuals, families, groups and communities are all levels of clients that can be assessed for specific needs and health risks. For instance, an individual might have an increased risk of reinfection from an unhealed wound following surgery. A family might have children at risk of malnutrition if the mother is not well informed about the benefits of a balanced diet and eating right. Populations might be at risk of a pandemic if vaccinations and immunizations are not taken seriously.

## Assess the client's readiness to learn, learning preferences and barriers to learning

As important as assessing the client is, if a nurse does not know the client's preferences and barriers, it can be very difficult to obtain cooperation.

Therefore, significant measures must be taken to understand clients, including how ready they are to learn, the best method for them to learn and possible barriers to their learning.

Readiness to learn is divided into four types:

A. Physical readiness: This involves the measures of ability, the complexity of the task, the effect of the environment, the health status of the individual and gender. The measures of physical ability determine if a patient is ready to learn or not. A patient that has a motor impairment might find it difficult to perform some fine movements and might not be ready to learn some things, such as cleaning a surgical wound appropriately. The complexity of the task must be proportional to the level of individual ability. The environment and health status can also affect an individual's physical ability to learn. A patient who is still drowsy and semi-conscious will not be ready to learn anything. A patient who lives in unfavorable conditions might not be ready to learn to live in a clean environment. Some studies have shown that the female gender usually displays more readiness to learn when compared to males. The reason is that women have traditionally picked up the role of caregiver and naturally pay more attention to things that pertain to health, either for themselves or family members.

B. Mental readiness: This deals more with the cognitive and psychological aspects of readiness. For example, a client who has just been diagnosed with a terminal condition might not be in a state of readiness to learn about it. The client might still be in shock or denial, and learning at this stage would be abortive. An anxious patient might also not be ready to learn because he or she might be unable to concentrate.

C. Experiential readiness: This deals with the levels of aspiration, coping mechanisms used in the past, the locus of control orientation and self-efficacy. Locus of control refers to the point where an individual's control or power over the future lies. In some people, the locus of control is internal; in others, it is external. When it is internal, then individuals believe that they have control over their own future and over any trouble they might encounter. When it is external, individuals believe that the future and whatever problems they might encounter are beyond their ability and lie in an external factor, like people.

The internal locus makes people more ready to learn. Self-efficacy is the belief individuals have that they can achieve a task or goal. It can either motivate or inhibit learning.

D. Knowledge readiness: Refers to the current level of knowledge of the learner, the level of capacity to learn and the preferred style of learning of the individual.

The style of learning varies from individual to individual. Some of the styles include visual learning, verbal learning, tactile (touch) learning, active learning, reflective learning and sequential learning.

Nurses should always combine multiple learning methods when educating several people at once. But when educating individual clients, they can utilize a person's most preferred learning method.

**Barriers to Learning**

The barriers to learning are many, and they depend on individuals, environments and teachers.

- Language barriers: Anyone who cannot communicate in English will need an interpreter or translator to communicate.
- Literacy level: When the literacy level of a client is low, the client might have difficulty reading and writing as well as understanding some technical words.
- Inadequate health information can also limit learning.
- Stress or pain can also be a barrier to learning, as the client might not be open physically or mentally to learning.
- Cultural and spiritual beliefs can be a major hindrance to learning, as they can make the individual close-minded to health facts.
- Physical and functional limitations such as disabilities or amputations can limit learning that requires physical movement.
- Financial limitations can also hinder learning. A client might be unable to pay for a procedure, training, class or needed materials.

## Plan or participate in community health education

Community health education refers to the study and development of health characteristics among target populations. It involves improving the personal, community and organizational health in society.

Nurses have to provide education to achieve these objectives of developing health characteristics. This involves assessing the particular health needs of a community. When these needs are identified, the nurse can devise a plan to intervene as needed. It might involve educating community members via presentations, counseling and guidance for individuals or even multidisciplinary cooperation. Regardless of the method, the nurse must be prepared at all times.

## Evaluate clients' understanding of health promotion behaviors/activities and educate them on actions

Health-promoting behaviors are actions that help increase individuals' health and well-being. Examples are exercise, a balanced diet, abstinence from smoking, abstinence from unprotected sex, avoiding drug abuse and illicit drugs, and receiving regular check-ups.

Assessing a client's knowledge of health-promoting behaviors can be done by asking questions. These questions can be informal but can provide an understanding of the client's level of knowledge.

Assessments can be structured and formal questions. They can also be made by observing the behavior of the patient. A patient who does not care about hygiene and does not wash his hands before eating might not be aware of the implications on his health.

Similarly, a client who does not bother about weight and continues to eat all types of junk food might either be ignorant or prefer to ignore the consequences of his actions.

Other assessment methods include focus groups, self-administered questionnaires, tests and documentation. Once the assessment has been done, educating the patient becomes straightforward.

**Weight management**

Patients can be guided to lose weight over a period of time in cooperation with a fitness coach, physical trainer and nutritionist. Clients can be educated about the complications of obesity and how it contributes to poor prognosis in many health conditions.

**Smoking cessation**

Patients often continue to smoke even though they know the negative effects of their actions. This can be due to addictions, depression and maladaptive coping mechanisms. Smoking cessation will require multidisciplinary cooperation with therapists, psychologists and physicians.

**Balanced diet**

A balanced diet helps to boost the body's immunity and ensure proper growth and development. When people do not eat well, their immunity breaks down. As a result, productivity, growth and even moods are affected. Nurses might need to collaborate with nutritionists to counsel clients on how to eat right. Patients with diabetes also benefit from this.

**Exercise**

Exercise is a health-promoting behavior. Clients should be counseled against a sedentary lifestyle. The WHO recommends at least 75 minutes of vigorous exercise every week and at least 150 minutes of moderate exercise weekly.

After educating the patient, follow-up is necessary to ensure that the therapies and education are productive. A follow-up helps to identify patients who need more help to achieve their set goals.

Apart from pharmacological and clinical interventions, some forms of treatment can effectively promote health. They include alternative and complementary therapies, such as meditation, prayers, chiropractic services, music, acupuncture or yoga.

## Educate clients about preventative care and health maintenance recommendations

A nurse's work also includes educating clients about routine recommendations to preserve health and prevent diseases. These include screening tests and regular routine examinations such as:

- Diabetes screening
- Cervical cancer screening in women
- Prostate cancer screening in men
- Colorectal cancer screening
- Hepatitis B and C screening
- HIV testing
- Hypertension screening
- Glaucoma screening
- Obesity education
- Breast self-examination
- Testicular examination
- Good nutrition/regular exercise
- Weight management
- Lifestyle choices such as cessation of alcohol, smoking and substance abuse

## Provide resources to minimize communication barriers

Communication is the exchange of information between at least two people. It involves the sending and receiving of information.

A barrier to communication is anything that prevents communication from happening.

Communication barriers can include:

- Language barriers: If clients do not understand English, they cannot understand what the nurse is saying. An interpreter that understands the client's language may be needed, or translation devices can be used if they are available.
- Physical communication barriers: Communication over wider distances and spaces can be easily misconstrued or misunderstood. Speaking to a large audience might not be very effective when trying to educate or counsel an individual patient.

   **Solution:** Nurses can leverage using wider audiences for general information and then ensure they have smaller breakout groups where the information is emphasized and opportunities are given for clients to ask questions. In some cases, one-on-one counseling might be required, as some individuals might be too shy to speak about their challenges in front of others. Different mediums should be explored depending on the information that needs to be shared.
- Physiological barriers: These are barriers that are due to the abnormal function of a body part, such as a hearing impairment or deafness. When this is the case, nurses should recommend a hearing aid for the patient or the use of sign language if the patient is completely deaf. If a person is blind, then Braille can be used in addition to speaking.
- Psychological barriers: Some patients might not be in a state of mind that is receptive to communication. A patient who just received a bad diagnosis might be shocked and depressed. A parent waiting for a child in surgery might be anxious. Patients might also have mental health conditions that do not make them open to communication.

   **Solution:** Nurses should understand the time or place for communication. If a patient or client is not in the best frame of mind and if the information is not urgent at the moment, it can be deferred until another time. If it is urgent, the nurse must be professional and empathetic while conveying the message. If it is a mental condition, then as treatment progresses, the client should be able to understand and receive information.

Other things to take note of in overcoming communication barriers include:

- Active listening: Nurses should listen to their patients carefully. People can tell if someone they are speaking to is listening or not.
- Clarity: Most clients do not understand medical jargon. Therefore, nurses should always speak in terms that patients can understand.
- Avoid information overload: The patients should be given time to take information in. The nurse is not the only person seeing the patients. Other health care personnel might be seeing them and giving them information. Therefore, patience is required so that clients do not get overwhelmed.

## Assist client in maintaining an optimal level of health

Nurses also have a role in helping patients to maintain an optimum level of health. An optimum level of health means the best possible level of health attainable by an individual based on their current health status.

For instance, a person who has had a limb amputated due to diabetes can still get to an optimal health status by regular blood sugar checking and complying with drugs. The person can use an artificial limb and crutch. A nurse can also collaborate with other specialists, such as physiotherapists, to help the patient learn to balance with the artificial limb or crutches.

Nurses can provide counsel on foot examination and prompt reporting to the health facility in case of any wound or break of the skin of the viable limb. They can provide counsel on wound care at the surgery site and the flap that was created at the amputation site. They can teach the client about signs of infection, such as pus, foul smell, discoloration or persistent bleeding.

# Lifestyle Choices

## Assess clients' lifestyle choices

Apart from the lifestyle choices that have been discussed in previous sections, some other choices greatly affect the health status of individuals. Some of these include the decision to either relocate to urban areas or stay in the suburbs, the decision to send children to schools or homeschool them and career decisions. All of these significantly affect the health status of individuals and families. For instance, a nurse can observe a difference when parents are around their children because they work remotely and have more flexible schedules than when they have to be out for most of the day. This can reflect in the bonding between kids and parents, more attention to their diet and growth and even their academics.

## Assess clients' attitudes/perceptions on sexuality

A nurse must be able to assess a patient's views and beliefs about sexuality. This includes sexual orientation, perception of gender, contraception, premarital sex, sexual partners and more.

Nurses must remain impartial and professional when relating to patients with different sexual orientations and perceptions, irrespective of what they believe.

## Assess clients' need/desire for contraception

Some clients might decide they do not need contraception. Nurses must be unbiased about the choices that each patient makes. They must share the benefits and disadvantages of different contraception types, including abstinence, withdrawal, calendar method, barrier method (male and female condoms, diaphragm, cervical cap), injectables, implants, intrauterine devices, female sterilization (bilateral tubal ligations) and pills.

## Identify contraindications to chosen contraceptive method

Some contraceptive methods have contraindications.

- Transdermal patches: History of smoking cigarettes, heart disease, deep venous thrombosis (DVT), breast cancer (or other estrogen-related cancers)
- Diaphragm: History of latex sensitivity
- Combined oral contraceptive pills (COCP): History of smoking cigarettes, heart disease, DVT, breast cancer (or other estrogen-related cancers)
- Emergency contraception: Pregnancy, vaginal bleeding
- Vaginal rings: History of smoking cigarettes, heart disease, DVT, breast cancer (or other estrogen-related cancers)

## Identify expected outcomes for family planning methods

Some of the expected outcomes of using contraceptives are:
- Ability to plan pregnancy
- Ability to prevent unwanted pregnancy
- Ability to have a satisfying sexual life without pregnancy concerns
- Ability to select the best methods of contraception based on needs and personal choices

## Recognize clients who are socially or environmentally isolated

When individuals are isolated, there are many implications for their health. It can result in depression, suicidal thoughts, low self-esteem and feelings of rejection. A nurse must be able to identify any individual who feels socially or environmentally isolated. This can be due to age, sickness, relocation of family members or death of a spouse.

Once the client is identified, interventions can be planned.

## Educate clients on sexuality issues

Clients must be educated on sexuality issues depending on the life stage they are in.

The major concern for those of childbearing age is fertility and family planning. Fertility can be an issue for either the man or woman. Infertility can be due to hormonal changes, infections, sexual dysfunction, trauma or surgery. Either way, there are medical advancements and tests that can help, including in-vitro fertilization and medical and surgical interventions.

## Evaluate alternative or homeopathic health care practices

The alternative health industry has been on the rise in recent years, with a surge in demand for natural remedies.

Homeopathy uses a natural approach to combat sickness and disease. While the effectiveness of some of the systems is not fully established, the FDA has concluded that they are safe.

# Self-Care

An ultimate self-care plan covers physical, emotional, psychological, spiritual, financial and environmental needs.

## Assess the clients' ability to manage care in the home environment and plan care accordingly

Assessment is a unique function of nurses. An ultimate self-care plan covers physical, emotional, psychological, spiritual, financial and environmental needs.

This plan encompasses looking out for basic activities of daily living that a client should handle upon discharge. Activities of daily living include personal hygiene, environmental sanitation, feeding, moving around, relationships with others, shopping, exercise, identification of certain medications to be used and so on.

Most times, patients being managed for mental disorders, certain illnesses or disabilities are assessed for their willingness and ability to care for themselves. Nurses check for physical strength, neurological balance, eye coordination and movement. They enforce the use of resources or aids to advocate for wellness and quick recovery.

For instance, a middle-aged man who was involved in an accident and lost the use of both lower limbs can be taught by the nurse how to care for himself. This will be done by assessment of the client's need for a wheelchair, assistance with moving around, bowel movement assistance and other means of caring for his body and oral health to maintain an acceptable level of functional independence.

Likewise, managing a client who just had a colostomy bag surgically implanted involves assessing for proper hygiene, monitoring personal intake and output, etc.

### Consider the clients' self-care needs before developing or revising the care plan

Clients' needs are unique, and nurses must approach them as such. Then an existing care plan can be modified based on need, or a new plan can be established.

For example, a plan to help a client manage bowel movements will differ from helping a client do a personal hygiene self-care review.

# Chapter 3: Psychosocial Integrity

Psychosocial integrity refers to equilibrium in the psychological and social areas of life. A nurse must be aware of factors that affect these areas, as well as how to intervene when necessary.

## Abuse or Neglect

### Assess clients for abuse or neglect and report, intervene and/or escalate

Abuse refers to any action in any form that intentionally causes harm to another person. There are several types of abuse:

- **Physical abuse:** This is the most recognized and involves any action that physically harms or injures another person, such as hitting, slapping, punching, confinement or isolation against a person's will, force-feeding and unauthorized restriction of movement.
- **Sexual abuse** refers to any form of sexual contact without consent. It can include unwanted touching, rape and forced nudity.
- **Emotional abuse** refers to causing emotional or mental pain deliberately.
- **Neglect** refers to depriving a vulnerable adult of basic or essential care needed to help maintain physical or mental health. Neglect can be due to actions or inactions, including failure to provide food, water, shelter, medications or access to health care.
- **Exploitation** refers to the illegal use of a vulnerable individual's resources for another person's profit. This can include illegally withdrawing money from a person's account, forcing a person to provide money or stealing items from a person.

The nurse must be able to identify signs of abuse.

Signs of physical abuse include bruises, black eyes, open wounds, untreated injuries, repeated visits to the hospital with injuries, lacerations, caregivers refusing to allow visits to the vulnerable adult, and reports of physical assault, among others.

Signs of sexual abuse include bruises around reproductive organs, vaginal bleeding that cannot be explained, shredded, stained or bloody undergarments, reports of sexual assault or rape and unexplained STIs.

Signs of mental abuse include personality changes, emotional agitation, anxiety around specific persons, reports of verbal or mental mistreatment, unusual behavior, withdrawal and nonresponsive behavior.

Signs of neglect include malnutrition and poor personal hygiene, bed sores from lying in the same position, reports of maltreatment, dirty clothing, unsafe and unhygienic living conditions and more.

Once these factors are identified, it is the duty of the nurse to report and plan interventions as appropriate.

**Identify risk factors for domestic, child and elder abuse or neglect and sexual abuse**

Some of the risk factors for abuse include:

- Older adults with cognitive impairment
- Children with developmental problems
- Mentally disabled people
- Physically disabled persons
- History of mental health disorders in the abuser
- History of substance use with the abuser
- Poor anger management skills of the abuser
- Crisis In the family or at work
- Female with no source of income or education

106

- Previous history of abuse

## Plan interventions for victims/suspected victims of abuse

Planning interventions can only be done after a thorough assessment of the patient's needs has been made. Once this assessment is done, the nurse should prioritize meeting the patient's needs.

The needs to be met depend on the presentation of the client. Patients that present with open wounds or injuries from battery should have their wounds attended to.

Those that are malnourished should be placed on a diet plan to supply appropriate nutrients. If a child is not feeling well, he or she should be nursed back to health.

Cases of abuse should be reported as the law requires.

The nurse must be able to establish an open, trusting and nonjudgmental relationship with the abused. Victims of abuse usually only open up when they feel safe and away from exploitation.

Nurses should be skillful at asking questions and be patient to get answers. They should also understand the time and place for some questions. A nurse might have to ask the caregiver/parent of a little girl to leave the room when she wants to ask some questions.

Intervention might mean taking the child into custody. The plan might also require multidisciplinary management, such as social health services, psychologists, counselors, physicians and nutritionists.

## Counsel victims/suspected victims of abuse and their families on coping strategies

Emotional support is required for individuals going through any form of abuse, and nurses are trained to provide just that.

Because of the cycle of violence and abuse, victims might feel like they need to go back to the abusive relationship. They usually need a lot of reinforcement and counsel on separating from the abuser to prevent the cycle from continuing. Doing this takes time and requires a lot of support.

The abuser needs to get help, such as anger management counseling. However, if the person has committed a crime, the law must be involved.

Abuse is a very serious issue and must be treated as such. It must be handled tactfully and professionally.

**Provide a safe environment for the abused or neglected client**

In the hospital, the abused should feel safe and secure. If the nurse observes anxiety in the patient when someone visits, then closer attention should be paid, and the visitor should not be allowed to see the victim without supervision (or possibly at all).

After discharge, abused children are usually moved from the home of the abuser to a different place that law enforcement authority will determine. Abused or neglected elderly can also be moved to facilities that will care for them better.

**Evaluate clients' responses to interventions**

After interventions are carried out, they should be evaluated. Was the wound well treated? Has the malnourished or dehydrated elderly patient begun to feed well? What is the client's current health status? Is the person adapting well to the new home they have been moved to? How well is the child coping with the situation?

## Behavioral Interventions

Behavioral interventions are designed in such a way that they alter the behavior of individuals on select issues. A nurse must understand how to identify patients that need this.

## Assess clients' appearance, mood and psychomotor behavior and identify/respond to inappropriate/abnormal behavior

Nurses can gauge a patient's psychological status by using appearance, mood and psychomotor behavior. These provide good insight into the mental health status of the individual.

From a patient's appearance, a nurse can tell if there are some possible conditions that might be present. A patient who dresses inappropriately for the weather, such as wearing thin clothing during the winter, might be struggling with a psychological or physiological issue. Additionally, the patient's gait, movement and grooming should be observed.

Mood can be assessed by observing both verbal and nonverbal communication. Is the mood appropriate for the occasion? A patient who begins to laugh after receiving the news of the death of a loved one definitely needs some attention.

Depression can present with low mood and loss of interest in previously enjoyed activities. This depressed mood can be reflected in the movement of the individual, which might be slow, with slumped shoulders and certain behaviors like avoiding eye contact.

Inappropriate behavior can be subtle or pronounced, or harmful to others. It is, therefore, the duty of a nurse to assess a patient properly and take proactive steps.

A patient who comes in drunk and staggering might be dangerous to themselves and others. A patient lashing out angrily can say things that upset other clients and health personnel.

A nurse should quickly inform security whenever she feels that the safety of any patient or personnel on the ward is at risk.

## Assist clients in developing and using strategies to decrease anxiety

Anxiety is the root of various inappropriate behaviors. Training clients to handle anxiety can be a very effective way to eliminate those inappropriate behaviors.

Some coping strategies include cognitive reframing, deep breaths, progressive relaxation, prayer, meditation, music therapy and medication.

## Incorporate behavioral management techniques when caring for a client

There are several techniques that nurses can use to help patients gain self-control over their behavior.

Examples of preventive measures include stress and relaxation techniques, avoiding identified triggers and stressors, use of consistent routines, exercise, alternative medicine, therapy and socialization activities.

If an episode begins, then the nurse might have to apply prompt de-escalation, maintaining eye contact while calmly and clearly asking the patient to desist from certain behavior, setting boundaries or using physical restraints as a last resort, especially when the patient can constitute a harm to themselves or others.

Other techniques that can be used include role modeling, in which nurses demonstrate appropriate and acceptable behavior around patients and staff members, and positive reinforcement, which involves acknowledgment and praise. Nurses should serve as accountability partners and provide support throughout the treatment.

Patient orientation is a program that helps to increase patients' sensory awareness and perceptions of reality.

Group therapy involves therapy with other people who have similar challenges. It can be grouped by age, sex, etc.

## Evaluate clients' responses to the treatment plan

The effectiveness of any plan depends on how well the patient has adhered to the structures and goals set.

These goals form the basis for the assessment of the treatment plan. Some common goals include the client demonstrating appropriate behaviors, identifying and avoiding triggers, sticking to boundaries and participating in required therapy sessions.

## Assess clients' reactions to the diagnosis and treatment of a substance-related disorder

Substance abuse is defined as the overuse of a substance that is addictive and/or not prescribed by qualified medical personnel.

Substance abuse can lead to physical dependence, which happens when a person begins to experience adverse physical reactions upon withdrawal of a drug. These adverse physical effects are usually more obvious when the drug withdrawal is abrupt. However, it is important to state that addiction can occur without physical dependence.

Addiction is the constant need for a person to take a particular substance despite obvious physical, mental and social or economic harm.

Psychological dependence happens when a person continues to use a substance to prevent any unpleasant feelings that occur if the substance is not taken.

## Assess clients for substance abuse and/or toxicities and intervene as appropriate

When clients are diagnosed, it is important for the nurse to observe them and their reactions. Some clients might be defensive, while others might feel ashamed.

Some clients might immediately admit their problem and then seek a way out. Others might blame others and rationalize their behavior. Some might present with low self-esteem masked with a buoyant personality or aggression.

Clients might have a low pain threshold, a high tendency to take risks or self-medicate, suicidal ideations and concurrent mental disorders.

Physically, there may be hyperactivity or sluggish movements, tremors, poor hygiene, the presence of needle marks on upper and lower extremities and poor health status.

Clients might exhibit drug-seeking behavior, such as claiming their medications have been exhausted, falsifying prescriptions and always having an ailment that requires medication.

They might also have problems in other areas of life, such as relationships, academics, social life and more.

Examples of standard tests for assessing such clients include:

- Drug abuse screening test
- Addiction severity index
- The CAGE-AID test
- Michigan alcohol screening test

**Plan and provide care to clients experiencing substance-related withdrawal or toxicity**

Substance-related toxicity occurs when a substance is taken beyond the therapeutic dosage at levels that constitute harm to the patient, and substance-related withdrawal symptoms occur when an individual cannot access a substance he or she has been abusing.

Some common signs of withdrawal and toxicity include irritability, restlessness, agitation, poor concentration, hallucinations and visual disturbances.

Some of the goals of care for patients with substance-related withdrawal or toxicity include:

- Safety and protection from self-harm and harming others

- Prevention of falls
- Relapse prevention
- Management of physical symptoms
- Ensuring medication is taken strictly as prescribed
- Educating the family and friends of the patient
- Introducing patients to self-help groups that can provide support during treatment

## Educate clients on substance use diagnosis and treatment plan

Once a plan is designed, the nurse is responsible for explaining and educating the client on the diagnosis, the treatment and the plans. The client's cooperation is essential to the success of the care plan. The patient should be educated on viewing the condition as an illness, not a defect, dealing with the stigma that is associated with substance and recognizing the risk factors that are associated with substance abuse.

## Provide care and/or support for clients with non-substance-related dependencies

Addictions are not limited to substances. There are non-substance-related addictions, such as sexual addiction, pornography addiction and kleptomania, among others.

For clients in this category, impulse control counseling and therapy could be useful. Cognitive-behavioral therapy and drug therapy can also be beneficial in addressing these disorders.

## Evaluate clients' responses to a treatment plan and revise it as needed

Evaluating a client's response is useful in determining if the client is progressing or suffering a relapse.

Some things to be considered include:

- Achieving sobriety
- Participating in therapy

- Responding to medication
- Attending support groups
- Understanding relapse and prevention mechanisms

## Coping Mechanisms

Coping mechanisms refer to patterns of behavior, thoughts and feelings that an individual uses to maintain a stable psychosocial status whenever there is stress or a disturbance. Stress can be due to many events, such as birth, death of a loved one, jobs or parenting.

### Assess clients' support systems and available resources

Different clients react to stress in different ways. A nurse must understand this while assessing them.

How people cope with stress is also affected by their environment and the type of people they surround themselves with. There are two standard assessment tools for this:

1. Interval Follow-Up Evaluation
2. Range of Impaired Functioning

### Assess clients' ability to adapt to temporary and permanent role changes

Some life events have temporary effects, while others bring permanent changes.

Temporary changes can include an injury or fracture that will take a few weeks or months to heal. They can also include the loss of a job, with the chance of obtaining another one later.

But permanent changes can include the loss of a loved one or a permanent lack of ability to perform at work.

Assessment is based on how people perceive their current status and the strategies they use to maintain their psychosocial homeostasis during the stressful period.

## Assess clients' reactions to a diagnosis of acute or chronic mental illness

Individuals react differently under stress. When the stress comes from acute or chronic illness, whether personal or that of a loved one, it can be very strenuous.

Some common psychological changes associated with acute or chronic illness include distress, anger, denial, guilt, grief, rationalization or depression.

## Assess clients' ability to cope with life changes and provide support

To better understand clients' perspectives and the various factors that affect their reactions, two models can be used:

- Social and cognitive models: These emphasize that clients should remain as independent as possible and be allowed to gain mastery over the situation rather than being pitied or looked down upon.
- Nagi model: This emphasizes that disability is a function of the social environment's expectations and the client's inability to meet them.

Support could include positive self-talk, social support systems, relaxation, stress management skills and helping the client to realign and readjust goals as necessary.

## Identify situations that may necessitate role changes for a client

Some roles in life come with serious changes that need some level of adaptation. Examples are newly established family units in young adults, new parents and caring for babies, middle-aged adults and health decline. Older adults may experience limitations in capacity and chronic illnesses.

## Provide support to clients with unexpectedly altered body images

When amputations or burns occur, clients can be affected to varying extents.

A disturbed or altered body image is confusion in the way clients view their physical body. When this image is impaired, it can lead to avoiding the use or hiding of the affected body part, negative feelings and remarks about the body or frequent referrals to past body image.

Interventions can include allowing clients to freely express their feelings about the alteration, facilitating the development of a more realistic body image and focusing on strengths and abilities rather than weaknesses.

## Evaluate clients' constructive use of defense mechanisms

Defense mechanisms are behaviors that people employ to avoid stress.

Some of these include:

- Displacement: This occurs when a client transfers anger, aggression or feelings of frustration at one person to another person or object.
- Regression: This occurs when a client is under extreme stress and begins to display behaviors that do not fit the person's current stage of development.
- Compensation: This occurs when a person succeeds extremely well in one activity or field in order to compensate for another area of failure.
- Intellectualization: This occurs when a person seeks to rationalize a stressful event in a way that makes it less painful or traumatic.
- Sublimation: This occurs when a client transforms unacceptable urges and feelings into socially acceptable urges.

Other defense mechanisms include dissociation, rationalization, undoing, identification or minimization.

## Evaluate whether clients have successfully adapted to situational role changes

If a client is adapting well and receiving treatment, there are some parameters to be checked:

- Coping with situational role change
- Realistic and achievable expectations
- Dependence on others
- Participation of family and friends in support and care
- Objective or subjective signs and symptoms

## Crisis Intervention

A crisis refers to a time-limited event that stresses an individual beyond the weight that a coping mechanism can handle.

There are different types of crises:

- Developmental/maturational crises: Predicted occurrences that happen in life. They occur due to growth (a new job or promotion at work), marriage, childbirth or retirement.
- Situational crises: Events that are unexpected and unpredictable. Examples are severe illnesses, job loss or the death of a loved one.
- Adventitious crises: Occur due to a major social disturbance, such as natural disasters, war or terrorism.

### Assess the potential for violence and use safety precautions

There are four main levels of crisis that a nurse must be able to assess for:

1. Level 1: Patients become anxious about life events and resort to coping mechanisms.
2. Level 2: Patients begin to show some signs of impairment or loss of function. To cope, clients begin to use different coping mechanisms from what they were using before.
3. Level 3: Patients begin showing signs and symptoms of typical general adaptation syndrome.

4. Level 4: At this stage, patients begin to feel isolated, detached and overwhelmed. Patients might begin to entertain thoughts of violence toward themselves and others.

Some risk factors for self-harm and violence to others include a history of depression, a history of self-harm, age greater than 45 years, past suicide attempts, non-heterosexual orientation and joblessness.

## Identify clients in crisis

Some things to look out for include saying goodbyes, oral or written suicidal statements, a loss of interest in activities once found pleasurable, changes in personality or appearance, changes in sleep patterns and self-harm.

Nurses should be able to pick any of these things up and use strategies to prevent violence or suicide.

## Use crisis intervention techniques to assist clients in coping

Any threats of suicide or violence should not be handled lightly. Patients can be placed on constant observation, and restraints can be used if necessary. But the first step is to establish trust with clients so that they can freely speak and express their feelings.

Then therapy can begin, and treatment will involve strong social support in the form of family and friends, who will provide positive reinforcement.

Clients should also be taught to develop their coping mechanisms and engage in individual and group therapy. Nurses should educate them about their conditions, how to identify signs of relapse and how to effectively reach out for help when needed.

## Guide the clients to resources for recovery from the crisis

Clients should be provided with resources about their condition and how they can be helped. Some of the outcomes to watch out for include decreased anxiety levels, effective coping mechanisms and seeking help.

# Cultural Awareness/Cultural Influences on Health

Culture is the way of life of a group of people. It refers to a set of established beliefs and ideologies that a group of people holds and which has been passed down from one generation to the next. A nurse must understand culture and its impact on how patients receive care.

## Assess the importance of clients' self-reported culture/ethnicity when planning/providing/evaluating care

Culture affects the way clients receive care. It affects how they perceive nurses and health care workers. A nurse must know how to relate to clients without offending their cultural beliefs.

Leininger's transcultural nursing theory proposes a model for both universal and specific nursing care. It proposes three nursing models that nurses must understand in order to provide care for people of different cultures:

- Cultural preservation and maintenance
- Cultural care negation and accommodation
- Cultural care repatterning and restructuring

These models provide a balanced approach to the assessment of culture and how it affects the delivery of care.

## Incorporate client cultural practices and beliefs when planning and providing care

Nurses must always ensure that they make allowance for their clients' cultural practices and beliefs whenever they are providing care. Many times this determines if the care will be received or rejected.

Some areas in which people hold different beliefs include:

1. Perceptions about health and sickness: Some cultures believe that ill health is a stigma, and therefore they distance themselves from it. Others promote health-seeking behavior, while still others do not believe in medical care; they believe in rituals and alternative medical practices.
2. A client might not readily receive intervention from a nurse. A nurse must patiently and tactfully introduce the concept of care. Such clients must not be rushed.
3. Family dynamics: The structures of families differ from culture to culture. Some cultures allow only males to make decisions about the family, including health matters. Others allow equal sharing of such responsibilities. Some cultures require the oldest member of the extended family to make decisions on behalf of other family members. A nurse must know who to approach when decisions are to be made.
4. Self-efficacy: Some cultures believe people can change their destinies or fate. Hence, they are willing to take steps to ensure that they get better or protect their health. Individuals with other cultural beliefs may not be so motivated to take steps because they believe the outcome all depends on fate.
5. Space and proximity: Some individuals are used to living in small towns with few people and might have difficulty adjusting to a busy hospital setting.
6. Cultures heavily influence communication patterns. This affects both verbal and nonverbal communication. A nurse might need an interpreter or translation device. A nurse must also be conscious of gestures, eye contact and signs which might be offensive to a patient.

Understanding these areas will help the nurse relate better with clients of different cultures.

## Respect clients' self-reported cultural background and practices

No matter how different a culture might seem, a nurse must respect all cultures as long as the particular beliefs do not harm any clients.

## Evaluate and document how client language needs were met

Documentation is part of the process of evaluation and growth. A nurse should document how client needs were met despite cultural differences and the techniques that worked. This not only helps the client to receive better care but also helps other nursing staff members to provide care in a way that the person understands.

Particular attention should be paid to the client's level of comprehension, compliance and adherence to care and treatments. Accommodations that can be made for such clients, such as the use of instructional materials, interpreters and translation devices, can also be documented.

# End-of-Life Care

End-of-life care can be challenging for everyone involved because of the physical, mental and emotional strain. However, nurses must remain calm because the clients need them to be at their best in periods like this.

## Assess clients' ability to cope with end-of-life interventions

A nurse must be able to assess the ability of a patient to cope with end-of-life interventions. A patient at this point has needs that are different from routine patients. They need physical, psychological, spiritual and physiological care.

Some physical needs might be adequate nutrition and fluids due to anorexia and dehydration. There might also be a need for pain medication.

Patients might have psychological needs. They might battle with confusion, sleep disturbances, fear and depression. These fears might result from different things, such as what will become of the family after they are gone, fear of the unknown and so on. Some of these issues can be corrected by the nurse, while others might have to be managed with the help of psychologists and family members.

### Assist clients in the resolution of end-of-life issues

End-of-life care should be adequately provided for clients that need it. In addition to what was mentioned earlier, this care might include proper hygiene, ensuring the patient is comfortable and providing privacy. It might also include proper turning and positioning of the patient at regular intervals, massage and therapy.

### Provide end-of-life care and education to clients

Nurses should educate clients about what to expect at this stage. The families and support system of the client should also be educated about the signs and symptoms to expect toward the end of life. It is very important that legal documents and advance directives be sorted out so that there are clear instructions on what to do and what not to do after death.

## Family Dynamics

There are different patterns that influence the outlook of life of family members, including their perspective on health care. The patterns determine how authority flows in the family, who makes the decisions, who is the leader and who is responsible for the care in the family.

### Assess barriers and stressors that impact family

Several barriers can impact the function of the family unit, including:

- Physical: Food, housing or transportation
- Biological: Ill health, disability or death
- Socioeconomic: Unemployment; lifestyle choices like drinking, smoking, substance abuse; underemployment; financial losses or war
- Cultural and spiritual stressors: Acceptance and rejection of culture by children, lifestyle choices

All these factors affect the function of the family in one way or another. Barriers such as lack of funds, lack of needed transportation and lack of cohesion in the family can all affect health care.

## Assess parental techniques related to discipline

Some parents are liberal, and others are very strict. Some go as far as abuse, and nurses have to be sensitive to know when a child is being abused. When violence is involved, nurses must report it to the appropriate authorities.

A nurse must observe all family members, especially the dependents, for any signs of depression, withdrawal or isolation, as these can all point to abusive behavior from the parent or caregiver.

## Encourage clients' participation in group/family therapy

Many families might not be open to family therapy. Nurses must be able to educate the family members on the need for group therapy and its benefits.

## Assist clients in integrating new members into the family structure

A new member of a family can be a stressor. This can be a problem in some families, especially if there are already some dysfunctions. A nurse can provide some education on what to expect from a new family member. In the case of a new infant, the parents and siblings should be prepared on what to expect and how to care for their newest family member.

## Evaluate resources available to assist family functioning

Once an assessment is made of the state of the family, then the nurse can come up with resources that can help the family unit. This can be anything from educational materials to resources in the community and referrals to qualified personnel who can provide therapy for the family.

## Grief and Loss

Grief is a normal response to loss that is characterized by emotional, physical, social and intellectual behaviors with the goal to eventually learn to accommodate or live with the loss.

Every loss will impact clients directly or indirectly, and the extent of grief that they exhibit will vary from person to person.

There are several types of grief, including:

- Dysfunctional grief
- Anticipatory grief
- Cumulative grief
- Collective grief

## Provide care for clients experiencing grief or loss

To properly provide care for a grieving patient, the nurse must understand the stages of grief. There are several theories with different stages.

The most popular theory is the Kübler-Ross model, which describes grief in five stages:

I.   Denial: This is when the person refuses to accept the loss that has occurred.
II.  Anger: This can be directed at oneself, the family, friends or the whole world.
III. Bargaining: This involves wishing things could return to what they were before the loss. It might also involve bargaining with a higher power if the event can be avoided.
IV.  Depression: This is when the person begins to really feel the loss. It is a crucial stage in healing.
V.   Acceptance: This involves living with the new reality that the person is gone.

Other models include Sander's phases of bereavement, which include shock, awareness of loss, conservation, withdrawal, healing or turning point and renewal.

Worden's four tasks of mourning include accepting the loss, coping with the loss, altering the environment to cope with the loss and resuming a healthy life.

Engel's stages of grieving involve shock and disbelief, developing awareness, restitution, resolution of the loss, idealization and outcome.

A nurse must understand what stage clients are in and help them accordingly. The first thing is to establish trust so that the client can be open to receiving help.

The nurse should also educate clients about coping strategies. There might be a need for referrals to social or religious groups. The services of psychologists might also be needed.

Standardized tools such as the Hogan grief reaction checklist and Texas inventory of grief can be used to assess clients for complicated grieving.

## Support clients in anticipatory grieving

Anticipatory grief begins before the event happens. It is usually seen in cases like terminal illnesses, loss or amputation of a body part.

The nurse can provide education on what to expect while being as gentle and empathetic as possible. But the facts should not be withheld or watered down, as this can negatively affect the client's expectations.

## Inform clients of expected reactions to grief and loss

Nurses should inform clients of what to expect while grieving. It might not be the happiest news to hear, but it helps to know that at least the nurse understands them.

## Evaluate clients' coping mechanisms and fears related to grief and loss

Clients must be evaluated to see how well they have coped with the grief and loss. They should be expressive about their feelings and not withdrawn or isolated, should seek help and have effective mechanisms to cope so they can resume their normal lives in one year or less.

If a client does not focus on anything else but the loss and cannot move beyond it, the patient might be experiencing complicated grief and require further help.

## Mental Health Concepts

Mental health is pivotal in treatment and care. Nurses must know about mental health disorders, how to assess them and what interventions are required.

### Recognize signs and symptoms of acute and chronic mental illness

A nurse must be able to recognize the signs and symptoms of a mental illness, whether acute or chronic.

Some mental illnesses include:

1. Depressive Mental Health Disorders: These include major depressive disorder, situational, developmental disorders, postpartum depression and others within this spectrum of disorders. Some tools for assessing this group of disorders include the Beck depression scale, the Geriatric depression scale and the Hamilton depression scale.

Signs and symptoms include low energy, depressed mood, loss of sleep, poor decision and judgment, weight loss, anorexia, loss of libido, personality changes, low self-esteem, hallucinations, delusions, suicidal ideation and suicide.

2. Anxiety Disorders: These include generalized anxiety disorder, different types of phobias, panic disorder, acute stress disorder, PTSD and obsessive-compulsive disorder. Tools for assessment include the Yale-Brown Obsessive-Compulsive scale, the Modified Spielberger state anxiety scale and the Hamilton Rating scale for anxiety.

Signs and symptoms can vary with specific disorders. Phobias present with anxiety or stress due to a particular object, event, location or situation. Panic disorders can present with chest pain, severe anxiety, difficulty breathing and palpitations. Generalized anxiety disorder can be present with persistent and prolonged worry over many things, and OCD may be present with pathological hoarding.

3. Bipolar Disorder: This presents with episodes of manic and hypomanic depression occurring at intervals. Signs and symptoms include elevated mood, irritability, depressed mood, restlessness, loss of inhibition, increased sexual drive, loss of sleep, grandiose delusion.

4. Cognitive Mental Disorders: This includes disorders such as dementia and delirium. Signs and symptoms include difficulty reading, poor writing and speech, inability to recognize people or places and poor short-term memory. Behavioral changes and impaired processes might also be present.

5. Personality Mental Disorders: These can be grouped into different clusters. Cluster A includes schizoid, paranoid and schizotypal mental disorders. Cluster B includes narcissistic, antisocial, histrionic and borderline disorders. Cluster C includes dependent and avoidant personality types. Signs and symptoms are dependent on the type of personality disorder. Cluster A personality disorders generally display odd or eccentric behavior. Cluster B personality disorders generally display dramatic or erratic behavior, while cluster C personality disorders are typified by anxious or inhibited behavior.

6. Eating Disorders: These include anorexia nervosa, bulimia nervosa and binge-eating disorders. Signs and symptoms include:

*Anorexia nervosa:* Excessive limitation of food intake, food binging or purging, extreme fear of weight gain, irritability, amenorrhea and low body weight.

*Bulimia nervosa*: Binge eating rapidly, followed by purging.

*Binge eating*: Repeatedly consuming large amounts of food at once.

7. Psychotic Disorders: These include schizophrenia, schizotypal personality disorder and schizoaffective disorder. Signs and symptoms include:

Cognitive symptoms such as poor attention and concentration, poor judgment and impaired decision-making. Affective symptoms include depressed mood, feelings of dejection and suicidal thoughts, hallucinations and delusions, lack of energy and motivation.

8. Substance Abuse and Addictive Disorders: These include alcoholism, sexual addiction and pornography addiction.

## Provide care and education for acute and chronic psychosocial health issues

Nurses are responsible for providing care for people with different behavioral health issues. Some of these issues might be acute, while others might be chronic.

The basis of providing care is the establishment of trust. Clients must be able to freely express themselves to the nurse. With this, a nurse can begin to provide the necessary care.

The care here would involve maintaining a safe, therapeutic environment for the client, administering prescribed medication, counseling and continuous observation of the patient's mental status by assessing behavior and providing education for the client and family members.

A nurse should educate the client and family members about the cause of the disorder, triggers and flashpoints, as well as about relieving factors, therapies, drugs, group therapy and follow-up care.

## Evaluate clients' ability to adhere to the treatment plan

Some clients might adhere to the treatment plan provided by the health care team, while others might not. The duty of a nurse is to evaluate the client's adherence to the plan.

Some of the parameters to look out for include the willingness and participation of the client in the plan, previous experiences where a similar treatment plan did not work, lack of insight of the client, the judgment of the client, denial, self-efficacy, internal locus of control and side effects of the plan.

## Religious and Spiritual Influences on Health

The influence of religion on a person can be powerful. Hence a nurse must understand how religion and spiritual beliefs affect health.

### Assess psychosocial factors influencing care and plan interventions

There are several psychosocial factors that influence the planning and delivery of care.

Occupational factors can include the nature of the job and the work hours. Some occupations may not allow patients the time to visit the clinic until weekends. Thus a nurse must create a flexible schedule for patients with such time constraints.

Other factors may pertain to remote workers who sit for long hours in front of a laptop. They must be educated on the need to have antiglare glasses and also take breaks regularly. They must also be counseled on the need to have a comfortable chair and working environment to prevent back pain or complications in the future.

Spiritual or religious factors play key roles in the planning and delivery of care.

There are many branches of Christianity, including Catholicism and Protestantism. Some Christians have beliefs about fasting, communion and newborn baptism.

Judaism also has different sects, some of which believe in circumcision, a kosher diet and death rituals.

Hinduism also has different philosophies and practices, such as yoga, a strictly vegetarian diet and death rituals.

Islam forbids pork and alcohol. Females may cover part of their faces. The body must be buried with white cloth at death.

Jehovah's Witnesses do not believe in blood transfusions, eating foods containing blood, abortion or suicide, among other things.

A nurse must attend to patients with a consciousness of their spiritual leanings and provide appropriate, respectful care for them.

## Sensory/Perceptual Alterations

Sensory and perceptual alterations usually occur at specific times, places and when the client is exposed to certain stimuli. Identifying the place where a patient is most vulnerable to these alterations can help prevent or reduce them.

A nurse should help the client develop coping mechanisms for these alterations or disturbances.

### Provide appropriate care for clients experiencing visual, auditory and/or cognitive alterations

Patients experiencing visual, auditory and cognitive impairments are at risk of inflicting harm on themselves and others. They can display aggressive or violent behaviors. Hence, appropriate care must be provided for them.

For patients experiencing auditory hallucinations, medication is usually the mainstay of treatment. Medication can also be combined with psychotherapy, education on coping mechanisms and cognitive-behavioral therapy.

Patients experiencing visual hallucinations usually have an underlying disorder such as schizophrenia. The underlying disorder should be treated, and medication can also be used. Cognitive-behavioral therapy and psychotherapy can also be useful for patients with this condition.

**Provide care in a nonthreatening and nonjudgmental manner**

Nursing care for patients with alterations or perception loss must be provided in a nonjudgmental manner, no matter what the clients are saying or the behaviors they display.

**Provide reality-based diversions**

Clients who are not oriented in time, place or person can usually be helped by creating reality-based diversions and activities. Activities include discussions and taking a walk.

## Stress Management

Homeostasis refers to a steady state of the body and its processes. It is a state of equilibrium and is what every system of the body strives to attain.

Stressors are factors that disrupt the equilibrium of the body. They can come in different forms, such as physiological, psychological, physical, emotional or spiritual.

Hans Selye proposed the general adaptation theory, which divides stress into three stages:

- Alarm
- Resistance
- Exhaustion

**Recognize nonverbal cues to physical and/or psychological stressors**

For nurses to effectively manage stress, they must be able to recognize nonverbal cues and respond appropriately. To do this effectively, nurses should understand the three stages of Selye's theory.

Alarm is the stage where certain physiological responses show that there is an upset in the body's homeostasis. Here, the patient might experience pupil dilation or increased heart rate, respiratory rate, glucose consumption, cardiac output and adrenaline and cortisol levels, with attendant manifestations. The goal of these manifestations is to prepare the patient to flee.

The resistance stage is marked by increased cardiac output, a maintained respiratory rate and increased blood pressure. Here, the body is trying to deal with the effects of stress. If it succeeds, the body will return to its normal resting mode. If not, then it continues in this resistance stage for a while before moving to the third stage.

The third stage is exhaustion. At this point, the body has used all its resources in trying to deal with the stress. If this stage is not reversed, morbidity and mortality may result.

A nurse must learn how to look out for the mentioned signs. Other signs to watch for include loss of consciousness, hyperglycemia and hypoglycemia.

### Provide information to clients on stress management techniques

A nurse should educate clients on different stress management techniques, which should include daily exercise, massage therapy, meditation and music therapy.

### Evaluate clients' use of stress management techniques

A nurse must evaluate how much progress is being made by clients in terms of stress management.

## Therapeutic Communication

Therapeutic communication refers to an exchange of information that occurs between patients and health care givers using both verbal and nonverbal cues in a manner that prioritizes the emotional and psychological well-being of clients.

### Use therapeutic communication techniques

A nurse must be able to use different means of therapeutic communication to reassure and counsel patients. Some of these techniques include:

**Active Listening:** This involves listening carefully to the patient, processing the information and observing the client's nonverbal communication.

**Silence** is a powerful tool of communication that, when properly utilized, can allow some time to process and deliberate before giving a response. However, this silence must not be for a prolonged period so that the client does not feel the nurse is not interested.

**Open-ended questions** help to get more information from the client and help the conversation flow better.

**Paraphrasing** is a good way for nurses to show that they are following a conversation. It helps to clarify things. For instance, "Do you mean that the pain you felt yesterday is not as severe as what you feel today?"

A nurse must be able to focus the discussion on the important issues at hand, even when the client wants to divert to other things not as pertinent at the moment. A client, for instance, might begin to discuss how he misses his pet. A nurse can respond, "Thank you so much for telling me about your pet. I am sure he can't wait to have you back. Now, let's discuss your hypertension and how we can deal with it together."

Other methods include clarification, which can be done by restating, paraphrasing and reflecting.

Nontherapeutic communication techniques to avoid include:

- Challenging: This means forcing clients to defend their choices and opinions.
- Probing: This is an invasive way of gathering information and is uncomfortable for clients.
- Changing the subject: This can be perceived as being rude or uninterested in what clients have to say.
- Defensiveness: This involves a nurse defending her own beliefs or opinions.
- Disagreeing with a patient: A nurse should try to educate clients in a therapeutic manner but not get into an argument with them.

- Judgments: A nurse must be nonjudgmental at all times.
- Stereotyping: This should always be avoided.

**Encourage clients to verbalize feelings**

Once trust is established between a nurse and a client, it becomes easy for clients to verbally express how they feel.

## Therapeutic Environment

Creating a therapeutic environment that facilitates and promotes the recovery of patients is essential to nursing care.

**Identify external factors that may interfere with client recovery**

Factors that can interfere with client recovery include family stressors, weak support systems, inaccessibility to quality health care and social stigma. Internal factors such as comorbidities and patient cooperation can also influence recovery.

**Make client room assignments that support the therapeutic milieu**

Assigning rooms to clients should be done in a way that supports the creation and promotion of a therapeutic milieu. A client who has suicidal tendencies, for instance, should be kept where nurses can observe the patient.

**Promote a therapeutic environment**

The goal of every nurse must be to establish and promote a therapeutically conducive environment for all patients. This type of environment is referred to as the therapeutic milieu.

Some of the elements of this type of environment include rules, boundaries, appropriate behavior, consistency and client expectations.

# Chapter 4: Physiological Integrity

Physiological integrity is divided into four components:

a. Basic Care and Comfort
b. Pharmacological and Parenteral Therapies
c. Reduction of Risk Potential
d. Physiological Adaptation

## Basic Care and Comfort

Basic care and comfort include assisting with activities of daily living. It includes assistive devices, mobility/immobility, nonpharmacological comfort measures, nutrition, oral hydration and postmortem care.

### Assistive devices

Assistive devices are equipment used to improve, augment and maintain an individual's performance and overall well-being. Assistive devices related to mobility and walking include walking canes, walkers, crutches, wheelchairs and prosthetic limbs. Some other devices, like alerting devices, sound amplifiers, electronic amplifiers and hearing aids, are designed to aid hearing loss. Patients with visual disabilities of any form may use corrective glasses (concave and convex) and magnifying glasses.

### Assess clients for actual/potential difficulty with communication and speech/vision/hearing problems

Basic care and comfort of patients begins with assessing communication, speech and visual acuity difficulty. Patients may have actual or potential speech, hearing and vision difficulties. Patients may need to be referred to an ophthalmologist and audiologist for further diagnosis.

Cerebrovascular accidents like a stroke can affect areas of the brain that deal with speech (speaking and understanding). These patients need a great deal of attention in addition to using assistive devices. People who are on medication like aspirin or other antibiotics that are ototoxic might eventually need assistive devices. These drugs damage the ear and present with initial symptoms of tinnitus and vertigo (ringing in the ear).

Elderly patients are also predisposed to macular degeneration in their eyes and this might result in total or partial blindness. Patients with chronic conditions like diabetes can end up with visual complications like blindness. Medications like antihistamines and antipsychotics can damage the eyes when overdosed. Nurses should know these types of patients and keep an eye on them.

**Assess clients' use of assistive devices**

It is nurses' responsibility to assess patients' use of devices, educate them on the correct use and correct the wrong use.

**Assist clients in compensating for a physical or sensory impairment**

A patient with a traumatic accident and a movement disability may need to use a walking cane. The cane should align with the patient's height for proper movement. The cane should be adjustable to permit the patient's elbow to flex slightly. The patient holds the cane opposite to the leg that needs support. For example, if the left leg is weak, the patient will hold the cane in the right hand.

Some other patients use wheelchairs. There are manual wheelchairs that need the patient to apply upper arm strength to move them or an assistant to push the chair. All of these assistive devices should be maintained and cleaned appropriately.

Patients may need special equipment to maintain their personal grooming. For example, patients may need adaptive hairbrushes, combs and special nail clippers. Also, oversized clothes, socks and zipper pulls may be helpful to some patients, along with certain kinds of toothpaste and toothbrushes.

Patients with assistive devices are prone to further accidents and injuries. Nurses should educate patients and their relatives on home care to prevent further complications.

## Elimination

Urinary elimination is a normal physiological process. After the ultrafiltration of plasma and selective absorption and reabsorption, urine must be eliminated from the body as it contains waste products, harmful metabolites and toxic substances.

### Assess and manage clients with alterations in bowel and bladder elimination

Urine elimination can be estimated in terms of quantity. A patient might eliminate above the normal reference range for a period of time. This is called polyuria. Polyuria can be caused by renal diseases, diuretic medication and diabetes mellitus. Other symptoms that can result from urine elimination quantity are oliguria, a reduction in urine output below the standard reference range for some time, dysuria, urinary incontinence, urgency and urinary frequency. These symptoms hint at pathology in the body and the urinary system.

Fecal elimination is also a normal physiological process. Fecal elimination follows the normal absorption of food and the digestion of food and nutrients. Pathologies that can affect fecal elimination include fecal impaction—the collection of hardened stool in the rectum. Constipation and some medications can also cause fecal impaction. Flatulence is the expulsion of malodorous gastrointestinal gas. Flatulence can result from foods or medication.

The knowledge of urinary and fecal elimination and their pathologies will help a nurse assess and manage patients with such illnesses. Some patients are highly predisposed to having urinary and fecal elimination problems. For instance, a patient on diuretics for heart failure or edema may have polyuria and an excess quantity of eliminated urine. Other patients who eat foods with high salt or sodium content may have reduced excretion of urine. Elderly male patients may have difficulty with urine elimination because of an enlarged prostate. For other patients, a structural defect or anomaly may be responsible for problems with urine and fecal elimination. It is also important to note that urine and fecal elimination is multifactorial—it can be structural, functional and even psychological.

Management of patients with urine and fecal elimination may require intervention by a nurse. Interventions like proper positioning during micturition and defecation are simple. Exercising to promote bowel movement is a simple intervention. Some patients only need privacy and comfort to empty their bowels and bladder. Food and diet also help to improve bowel movement and fecal elimination. Foods like boiled lentils, black beans and split peas contain high fiber and help promote bowel function.

Medical management of elimination problems includes using pharmacological agents to relieve elimination problems. It is usually attempted before surgical interventions. Medication can improve urine elimination. Such medications include oxybutynin and darifenacin. Enemas are also examples of medical management of conditions like constipation. Enemas are injectable fluids used to stimulate the emptying of the bowels. They can also treat fecal incontinence and flatulence.

Urinary catheterization is a minor surgical procedure to relieve urinary retention and empty the bladder. Nurses should be careful with this procedure as it can introduce microbes directly into the genital tract if not aseptic. Once the catheter is placed in situ, the nurse should ensure that the urine bag is emptied as necessary. Another form of surgical management is colostomy. A colostomy is a surgical procedure to heal anastomoses, relieve bowel obstruction and eliminate fecal content. There are different types of colostomies, all with a similar goal of allowing proper elimination.

The overall aim of these interventions, whether therapeutic, medical or surgical, is to restore and improve the elimination capacity of the urinary and rectal tracts.

**Evaluate whether clients' ability to eliminate is restored/maintained**

Restoration of elimination function and capacity is accompanied by the ability to perceive voiding clues. Also, the patient will be free of symptoms like urinary urgency, frequency and pain. The absence of diarrhea and constipation is a sign of restored eliminating function. Patients who show positive signs of restoration of normal urinary or bowel functions may be evaluated and possibly discharged.

## Mobility/Immobility

Nurses should understand why and how immobility can occur in patients.

### Assess clients for mobility, gait, strength and motor skills

Mobility is the ability to move freely and with purpose. The first skill a nurse should have in managing patients with potential immobility is assessing gait and movement. Just like most disease conditions, risk factors predispose people to stiffness. These factors can be genetic or acquired. Genetic factors can be cognitive impairment and spasticity. Other genetic factors include the natural weakness of the bones and muscles. Some other patients acquire immobility due to medication use, overdose, malnutrition, impaired gait and trauma.

When a nurse identifies patients with these risk factors, the next step is to assess for actual immobility. Assessment of mobility begins with observation. For instance, a patient with a weak gait could become immobile. Nurses can also assess immobility in a patient by giving simple instructions. For instance, ask the patient to move on the bed or around it. Assessment of mobility also involves the time it takes for the patient to get up from the seat. The ability to sit on a chair and stand is also part of the mobility assessment.

Mobility is multifactorial. The nerves, muscles, electrolytes and psychology all come together to ensure proper mobility. Any of these can be affected so mobility is compromised. Muscle contraction—one of the parameters that determine proper mobility—can be assessed and scored for each patient. A patient is scored from 0 to 5.

**Identify complications of immobility**

The complications of immobility are systemic, affecting not only the muscular system but also the urinary, gastrointestinal and respiratory systems.

When the respiratory muscles in the airway are immobile and cannot expel secretions, this can lead to respiratory infections, atelectasis and hypostatic pneumonia. Shallow respiration and decreased respiratory movement are also complications of immobility.

When urinary muscles cannot expel urine, there is urine retention and stasis. Stasis and urine retention predispose a patient to the formation of renal stones and the development of urinary tract infections.

The gastrointestinal system is also affected by immobility. Bowel movement is reduced. The patient can present with constipation, impaction and difficulty with evacuation.

Immobile skin can break down and lose its turgor. The skin of immobile patients ulcerates and loses its strength.

Lastly, the musculoskeletal system suffers greatly from immobility. The muscles, bones and joints become very weak. The bones can suffer from osteoporosis and hypocalcemia. There's a higher risk of bone fractures. The joints can become stiff and very painful. This can further limit the range of motion of the patient.

**Evaluate clients' responses to interventions to prevent complications from immobility**

For the urinary and gastrointestinal systems, the nurse should ensure adequate fluid intake. Fluid intake eases and helps bowel and bladder movement. Regular exercise can stretch weak muscles, bones and joints. Also, the patient should engage in deep breathing and coughing to clear the respiratory system of secretions.

**Perform skin assessment and implement measures to maintain skin integrity**

The skin is the body's first line of defense. So, it must be well assessed for color, odor, drainage or exudates, texture distribution and margins.

The best way to maintain the integrity of the skin is to prevent a breakdown in the first place. Steps to take to prevent the breakdown of the skin include:

- Screening of clients for possible skin breakdown on a regular basis.
- Keeping clients always clean and dry to prevent the buildup of moisture.
- Balanced diet and adequate fluids to keep clients well-hydrated and nourished.
- Using devices like wedges, pressure-relieving mattresses (waterbeds) and pillows to prevent bed sores from friction and pressure.
- Regular turning patients who cannot turn independently.
- Identifying those clients at risk of pressure ulcers. This can be done using screening tools such as the Braden scale.

**Apply, maintain or remove orthopedic devices**

Orthopedic devices serve various purposes in skin and musculoskeletal care. Some of the most common are:

- Traction: Traction uses physical forces to exert pressure on a body part. It includes skin traction, skeletal traction or manual traction.
- Splints are used in fractures of the limb to prevent further damage to the soft tissues.
- Braces are used to provide support to body parts.
- Casts are used to immobilize body parts when a fracture has occurred.

**Implement measures to promote circulation**

Measures to promote circulation include the use of anti-embolism stockings and compression devices. They also include range of motion exercises, positioning and repositioning workouts and routine exercise and mobilization. The goal of all these activities is to prevent the formation of clots, encourage smooth blood flow and increase overall well-being. Some of these workouts also improve mental health and balance.

## Nonpharmacological Comfort Interventions

Interventions and therapy can be medical (pharmacological) or nonpharmacological. While it is crucial to know pharmacological therapy, foundational knowledge of nonpharmacological therapy is also essential.

**Assess clients for pain and intervene as appropriate**

Before these interventions can be applied, patients must be assessed and diagnosed.

Acute pain is a classification of pain based on a duration of less than three months. It is rapid in onset, localized and most likely severe. Chronic pain, on the other hand, is extended. Some pain is deep in the body and some is superficial.

**Recognize complementary therapies and identify potential benefits and contraindications**

There are many nonpharmacological interventions that have potential benefits. Some are complementary, alternative or integrative modalities. They include meditation, magnets, prayer, homeopathy, chiropractic services, acupressure, massage and guided imagery.

Some indications for these services are chronic lower back pain, stress, neck pain, depression and fibromyalgia.

Some contraindications to chiropractic services are spinal cord compressions. Clients with pacemakers or insulin pumps should avoid magnets.

**Provide nonpharmacological comfort measures**

Nonpharmacological comfort interventions begin with education about the patient's pain. Other comfort interventions include companionship, exercise and massage. Distraction from their current medical condition can work well for children. Counseling sessions, drama, art and music are some other interventions that are nonpharmacological.

## Nutrition and Oral Hydration

Nutrition plays a significant role in health.

### Evaluate clients' nutritional status and intervene as needed

Assessment of patients' nutrition can be done by collecting data. This data will include height, weight, body mass index (BMI) and waist circumference. Other data, including laboratory values of essential chemicals like hemoglobin, lipid and protein in the body, will reveal excess or reduced values. The nurse should also ask patients about their daily diet.

Managing patients with nutritional problems depends on the patient's condition. Patients with obesity should be put on a weight reduction regimen. This may include changes in diet habits and light exercises. Patients recovering from a physical disease might need to gain weight. Such patients can be put on supplements.

### Provide client nutrition through tube feedings

Tube feeding is also known as enteral nutrition and it involves passing tubes from the nose to the stomach or intestine. Clients who require tube feeding are typically those with gastrointestinal disorders, swallowing problems, burns or any other condition that results in an inability to obtain adequate calories or nutrients through oral ingestion.

Tubes can be placed either noninvasively or invasively, although noninvasive tubes are preferred. Noninvasive tubes require a good gag reflex and swallowing ability.

Clients should be seated 30 degrees upright. Tube feedings can be given either on a continuous, intermittent or bolus basis.

Tube placement can be confirmed by radiography, auscultation or pH of aspirate. Input and output should be monitored, and securing tape should always be used. The nurse should also watch out for signs of irritation, infection or dislodgement.

**Evaluate client intake and output and intervene as needed**

Intake refers to all the foods that are consumed by a patient, including IV fluids and feeding via tubes. Output refers to the elimination of food and fluids from the patient's body. Both solid intake and output are also measured. Urinary output and liquid stools are also measured.

Deficits should be corrected by increasing fluid intake either through oral means or intravenously. Fluid loss should be minimized where possible.

## Personal Hygiene

Personal hygiene is the most basic care that individuals can give themselves.

**Assess clients' performance of activities of daily living and assist when needed**

Personal hygiene should be done daily. The role of a nurse in ensuring personal hygiene includes education and assessing patient's hygiene.

Personal hygiene starts with bathing to cleanse the body of dirt, sweat and chemicals. Nurses can bathe patients who are in the hospital. The water temperature must be checked and soap must be available.

Other aspects of personal hygiene include perineal care, where the skin of the perineum is cleaned and washed regularly to avoid infections and odors. Shaving is also a part of personal hygiene. Oral hygiene involves brushing the teeth twice a day and rinsing the mouth. Caring for nails and feet is also part of personal hygiene.

**Performing Postmortem care**

After a client's death, all medical equipment should be removed, such as any catheters or IV lines. The entire body of the deceased is washed and limbs are placed in proper alignment. Eyes and mouth are shut and the patient is wrapped in a shroud. The body should be identified before being transported to the morgue.

## Rest and Sleep

Insomnia is the inability to sleep. It is multifactorial. Insomnia can be a result of medication that causes sedation. It can also be caused by the environment, illnesses, emotional and psychological disturbance and lifestyle.

### Assess clients' sleep/rest patterns and intervene as needed

Nurses can assess their patients for sleep patterns. For instance, a patient who drinks alcohol may have a disturbed sleep pattern. It is also essential to record sleep patterns, such as how long the patient slept and the duration of sleep.

# Pharmacological and Parenteral Therapies

Pharmacological and parenteral therapies involve medications that are taken both orally and through other routes of drug administration. Nurses administer medication orally, intravenously and intramuscularly. Parenteral drug administration refers to any non-oral method but usually involves injecting directly into the body, bypassing the skin and mucous membranes. Medication is a big part of the treatment regimen for many disease conditions. The knowledge of pharmacology, medication side effects and allergies will be helpful for every nurse.

### Adverse Effects/Contraindications/Side Effects/Interactions

Medication administration requires the nurse to use critical thinking abilities, professional judgment, pathophysiology and detailed knowledge of patients and their condition.

Before administering medications, the nurse must be thoroughly informed of the medications' contraindications and the patient's condition. Some general contraindications to medications include pregnancy, allergy to the medicine and renal disease. These patients will need special considerations during drug administration and treatment.

Some drugs interact with other medications. Due to this, nurses must be careful when administering multiple medications.

Some patients are allergic to certain medications. For example, some patients react negatively to medication containing sulfur. Some patients are also allergic to penicillin and antibiotic drugs called cephalosporins. Allergic reactions to drugs vary from moderate to severe and life-threatening. Nurses must assess patients to detect the possibility of reactions to medications. The signs and symptoms of allergic reactions can range from itching, body rash, swelling and redness to reduced blood pressure, respiratory distress and rapid pulsation.

Nurses who assess that a patient has had a severe side effect or adverse consequence from medication or parenteral therapy must record this information immediately. The patient should stop taking the drug until the doctor who prescribed it responds with further instructions.

### Blood and Blood Products

Blood is a body fluid that contains plasma and blood cells. The blood cells include red blood cells, white blood cells and platelets. Blood has significant oxygen functions and transports nutrients. It is responsible for clot formation (to prevent blood loss), fighting infections and regulating body temperature.

Blood products are therapeutic substances derived from blood. The different blood products and their components are made of red blood cells, platelets, fresh frozen plasma, albumin, clotting factors, cryoprecipitate and whole blood. Blood cells, especially red blood cells, have antigens. A blood type has A antigens; B has B antigens; AB has both A and B antigens and O has neither A nor B antigens.

Individuals with blood types A, B, AB and O can receive type O blood, but only individuals with type O blood can receive type O blood. Patients with type O blood are universal donors but not universal receivers. Each blood type also contains antibodies, sometimes known as agglutinins. B agglutinins are present in type A blood; A agglutinins are present in type B blood; no antibodies or agglutinins are present in type AB blood; and A and B agglutinins are present in type O blood.

Patients with hypovolemia brought on by bleeding, anemia or other conditions involving a deficiency in coagulation or another blood component are advised to receive blood transfusions. However, people with certain religious beliefs will not accept blood transfusions.

**Administer blood products and evaluate clients' response**

Before a blood transfusion, the nurse must crosscheck if the patient is the right patient. A catheter must be inserted and an intravenous line (either central or peripheral) must be attached. When administering blood or a blood product, the nurse must closely watch the patient for signs and symptoms of a potential problem. When a reaction or complication is possible, the nurse must immediately halt the blood or blood product delivery.

Some complications associated with blood transfusion include febrile reactions, hemolysis, allergic reactions and sepsis. The most common reaction to blood and blood product administration is a febrile reaction. Although a febrile response can occur with any blood transfusion, it is most commonly linked with packed red blood cells and is not followed by hemolysis. This transfusion reaction is characterized by fever, nausea, anxiety, chills and warm, flushed skin.

ABO incompatibility, which results in hemolysis, is an incompatibility between the recipient's and donor's blood types. This incompatibility may result from a practitioner error while examining the blood and matching it to the patient's blood type and a laboratory error regarding typing and crossmatching. The presence of flank discomfort, chest pain, restlessness, oliguria or anuria, respiratory distress, brown urine output, hypotension, fever, low blood pressure and tachycardia are signs of this condition. Hemolysis is treated by administering normal saline once the transfusion is discontinued and changing all tubing to prevent kidney failure and circulatory collapse.

A blood transfusion may also cause a mild-to-severe allergic response. A blood plasma protein allergy often causes a mild allergic reaction, but a significant antibody-antigen interaction usually causes a severe one. Itching, pruritic erythema, swelling of the lips, tongue or pharynx, as well as flushing of the skin, are symptoms of mild allergic reactions. Chest pain, low oxygen saturation, unconsciousness, flushing, shortness of breath and respiratory stridor are symptoms of severe allergic reactions. Corticosteroids and antihistamine drugs are used to treat mild allergic reactions, whereas supplemental oxygen and pharmaceuticals are used to treat severe allergic reactions.

**Central Venous Access Device**

A central and peripheral venous access device can be used for venous access. When patients have accessible and usable veins, peripheral intravenous devices are utilized for short-term intravenous therapy, including fluids, electrolytes, medicines and chemotherapy. Various factors should be considered when choosing a vein for a peripheral intravenous device. The distal veins on the nondominant hand are the ideal choice so the client can fully use the dominant hand. A mastectomy side, the side of paralysis or a dialysis access device are not used.

Locations distal to past phlebitis or infiltration sites should be avoided. Hand veins are not the veins of preference. The upper extremities are used whenever possible, rather than the legs, to avoid lower extremity phlebitis and embolism.

Inserting a peripheral intravenous catheter begins with locating a suitable vein and positioning the tourniquet three to four inches above the vein on the patient's arm. After cleaning the area with an alcohol swab, have the patient create a fist. Insert the catheter into the vein at a 15- to 30-degree angle. When blood flashes back into the catheter, remove it. Secure and stabilize the catheter with care. Monitor and maintain the intravenous line and the insertion site after the catheter is implanted to ensure it is patent and the flow rate is as specified. Examine the intravenous site for symptoms of infection and infiltration.

## Access and/or maintain central venous access devices

Central venous catheters are placed into the right atrium of the heart via the superior vena cava. They can be introduced into the superior vena cava via a peripheral vein, as with a peripherally inserted central venous catheter (PICC), or via the subclavian or jugular vein. Central venous catheters are the preferred method of gaining venous access when a patient is receiving intravenous fluids or treatments at home, when there are insufficient peripheral veins for the patient's needs or when the patient is receiving therapy such as total parenteral nutrition, chemotherapy, blood and medication.

Infection, pneumothorax, hemothorax, thrombosis and emboli are some risks connected with central venous catheters.

When central venous lines are set, nurses must provide extra care for such patients. Central venous catheters should be changed every 48 hours, and each catheter's lumen should be flushed with heparin daily to ensure the patency of the tubes.

## Dosage Calculations

Nurses administer medications and must know how to calculate the correct dosage to avoid drug overdose.

## Perform calculations needed for medication administration

Calculation of medication dosages can be pretty technical. There are different methods for measurement and calculations. Units of measurement might differ, but a nurse should know some standard measurements. Here are a few examples:

1 teaspoon = 5 ml

1 tablespoon = 15 ml

1 cup = 16 tablespoons

1 pound = 12 ounces

1 scruple = 20 grains

1 pint = 16 ounces

1 quart = 2 pints.

10 centimeters = 1 decimeter

Numbers can be written as fractions or mixed numbers. Fractions can be proper or improper. The number on top is the numerator, while the number below is the denominator.

Mixed numbers are a combination of whole numbers and fractions. They should be converted to improper fractions before they can be used in calculations.

Decimals are expressed using a decimal point.

These forms of measurement are converted from one to the other. For example, when a doctor recommends a prescription in grains (gr) and you have the medication, but it is measured in terms of milligrams (mg), you will need to convert between the two measurement systems.

Calculating doses and solution rates requires nurses to use their clinical judgment and analytical skills. A nurse should be able to see an inaccurate calculation right away. Accuracy is vital in pharmacological measures because it can affect the patient's treatment. For example, medication for pediatric patients needs extra accuracy in dosage, routes and concentration.

**Expected Actions/Outcomes**

Nurses anticipate outcomes from the treatment regimens of patients.

**Evaluate clients' use of medication over time**

In a world where change is constant, nurses provide continuous care. The number of new medications, side effects and outcomes has grown to the point where it is impossible to remember them all. As a result, nurses administering medication must be knowledgeable about their patients' health concerns and the complexities of the medicine they use, using problem-solving, clinical decision-making and critical-thinking skills.

Some patients take pharmaceuticals for a short time for an acute sickness, whereas others are given medications for an extended amount of time for a chronic health issue. Prescription pharmaceuticals, over-the-counter medication, vitamins, supplements and alternative medications are examples of these medications.

**Evaluate client responses to medication**

Nurses caring for patients on multiple drugs for an extended period must keep track of the patients' adherence and compliance with their drug schedules. They must also assess the medication's predicted outcomes. Nurses must closely watch for adverse reactions, interactions or undesirable effects. They must monitor patients for evidence of any accumulated effects of the drugs they've taken over time.

The term "side effects" refers to all consequences of a drug that are not the expected or desired therapeutic impact of the medication. Some side effects can be significant. An adverse effect is a severe side effect that can sometimes be fatal, such as an allergic reaction to a medication.

**Medication Administration**

Medication administration is a cardinal aspect of nursing care and patient treatment.

## Educate clients about medications

Before medication administration, the patient should be informed about the medication, its expected effects and potential side effects. Patients, as well as significant partners, should be educated on all aspects of their drugs.

## Participate in the medication reconciliation process

The patient should know how and where the drug should be safely stored. The nurse should explain the significance of verifying the medicine's label for its name, dose, expiry date and the method for administering it. Particular directions should be provided, such as shaking the drug, taking it with or in-between meals or on an empty stomach.

## Handle and maintain medication in a safe and controlled environment

Some patients may need to administer medication at home. The patient should be instructed on how to self-administer drugs properly. In addition to the instructions outlined above, some patients may need to be trained on unique procedures such as using an inhaler, mixing insulin, giving oneself an intramuscular injection or self-administering tube feedings.

Routes of drug administration include oral, sublingual, topical, transdermal, inhaled and intravenous. The oral route of drug administration is the most common, most accessible and most convenient for patients. The intravenous route has 100 percent bioavailability. This means that all the medication administered into the veins will reach the target organs.

## Evaluate appropriateness and accuracy of medication orders for clients

Nurses are responsible for reviewing every order to determine its accuracy and appropriateness relative to the patient in question.

Some of the factors to be considered include the completion of the medical order, accuracy of the order, any client allergies, the health status of the client and significant laboratory findings.

## Pharmacological Pain Management

Pain alerts the nervous system that something is amiss. It is a sensation such as a prick, tingle, sting, burn or aching.

### Administer medications for pain management

Nurses help manage pain by administering medication to patients. The level of pain and type of pain will determine the medication dosage and the strength of the pain medication.

Analgesics are pain medications. They are broadly classified as weak, moderate or strong. Opioids (narcotics) are used to treat moderate-to-severe pain. Non-opioids are non-narcotic analgesics that can be used as adjuvant painkillers in addition to treating mild pain. Nonsteroidal anti-inflammatory drugs (NSAIDs) are examples of non-opioid drugs.

### Handle and administer controlled substances within regulatory guidelines

It is necessary that nurses follow the required guidelines when administering controlled substances because of the prevalence of addiction and substance abuse. Some of these guidelines include:

- Signing before receiving medication.
- Delivering the narcotics sheet to the nursing care unit along with the drugs.
- Locking drugs in secure locations.
- Counting narcotics at the start and end of every shift.
- Signing upon removal of any controlled substances from the locked cabinet for administration to clients.

## Total Parenteral Nutrition

Stronger immune systems, safer pregnancies and deliveries, a decreased risk of noncommunicable diseases (including diabetes and cardiovascular disease) and longer life spans are all associated with proper nutrition.

### Administer parenteral nutrition and evaluate client response

Total parenteral nutrition, known as hyperalimentation, is administered through a prominent vein, such as the subclavian vein. Hyperalimentation can meet all dietary requirements, with feedings containing minerals, electrolytes, vitamins, amino acids and trace elements supplied via the hyperalimentation catheter, which the physician surgically implants.

Total parenteral nutrition is most often used for patients who require complete bowel rest, those in a negative nitrogen balance due to a severe burn or another cause and those with a serious medical illness or disease such as cancer or AIDS/HIV. Total parenteral nourishment is given in the same way that intravenous infusions are.

## Reduction of Risk Potential

Reduction of risk potential is an important skill every nurse should have. It reduces the likelihood of clients developing complications or health problems related to existing conditions, treatments or procedures.

When nurses attend to patients for a particular condition, complications may arise from disease conditions or the treatment modality. Complications are the final results of disease conditions or treatment regimens. They can alter the recovery process of patients and lead to constant changes in the treatment regimen of patients.

Causes of complications are multifactorial. They may arise from a weak immune system or late presentation to the hospital. Complications may arise from inadequate dosing or improper monitoring of the treatment process.

Some of these factors are beyond the nurse, but nurses must make the treatment process as standardized as possible.

## Changes/abnormalities in vital signs

A patient's vital signs reveal much about the recovery process, status or underlying medical conditions. A nurse should be able to assess and respond to changes in a patient's vital signs. A patient's vital signs include blood pressure, pulse rate, respiratory rate and body temperature. These four signs signify the body's most basic function. For example, a consistently high body temperature in a three-year-old child is cause for concern.

Knowledge of the anatomy of the body and the pathophysiology of diseases is critical in noticing and responding to abnormal vital signs. For instance, knowledge of anatomy helps a nurse read the radial pulse on the lateral side of the wrist. The nurse puts the cuff around the arm to measure blood pressure. The nurse listens to the Korotkoff sounds over the cubital fossa with a stethoscope. Blood pressure readings also reveal much about what is happening to the heart. The systolic pressure indicates the force the heart pumps blood out with and how much resistance it is overcoming.

Assessment of the respiratory rate starts by inspecting the rising and falling of the chest. An unexplained increase or decrease can be a sign of pathology in the body. For example, a decreased respiratory rate can indicate central nervous system depression. A patient who presents a reduced respiratory rate may be an opioid drug user or may have recently been overdosed with sedative drugs, which depress the central nervous system.

## Diagnostic tests

Investigations are the second line of assessment in diagnosing and treating diseases. A nurse should be able to perform basic diagnostic tests. These tests reveal an accurate picture of what is happening to a patient. They also help caregivers arrive at a diagnosis and the appropriate treatment regimen.

Diagnostic tests can be invasive and non-invasive. Nurses should be able to do non-invasive diagnostic tests like blood glucose monitoring and electrocardiogram. Before starting any test, it is necessary to confirm the doctor's order for the tests and that the right patient is getting the proper test.

The testing kits and equipment should be by the patient's bedside to start any diagnostic test. The nurse should do a brief introduction of the whole process. The patient must give consent to the test before proceeding. Proper handwashing before and after the test is essential to keep the process aseptic. Afterward, the nurse should dispose of used equipment appropriately.

Blood glucose monitoring is a noninvasive procedure. The nurse should use the right strip and meter. The patient's finger is cleaned with an alcohol swab to disinfect it. A rapid needle prick is done on the side of the finger using a lancet. Turn the finger downward to allow the blood to flow. Wipe off the first drop of blood with a sterile gauze and collect the next drops of blood on the strip. To stop the blood, apply pressure over the puncture site with sterile gauze until the blood stops flowing. Then read the blood glucose level. Blood glucose level is essential in managing patients with diabetes.

Similarly, the electrocardiogram (ECG) is a noninvasive diagnostic test that traces the heart's electrical activities. It involves leads placed on the exposed chest, hands and leg. Then the activities of the heart are read on an electrocardiograph.

**Laboratory Values**

Some diagnostic tests require comparing the patient's test values to the standard laboratory or reference value. Laboratory tests are necessary to assess the levels of chemicals, hormones, enzymes, waste products and even markers in various body fluids and specimens.

Specimens collected for laboratory testing include blood, urine, feces, semen, saliva, semen and other body tissues. Collection of these samples requires skill, practice and proper knowledge. These tests can frighten some patients, especially pediatric patients who might fear needles and syringes. The nurse should explain the process to the patient like any other test and obtain consent.

Blood samples can be collected in three ways; arterial sampling, venipuncture sampling and finger prick sampling. Venipuncture is the most common way to collect blood from an adult patient. The collection of blood is from a superficial vein in the upper limb where the vein is easily accessible. The skin is cleaned with an alcohol swab, and the arm is tied with a tourniquet to make the veins more visible. A cannula is introduced into the vein slowly and blood is collected into a bottle.

Venipuncture is the process of collecting blood from veins. It is a relatively safe procedure but can also have complications for both the patient and the nurse. The patient is at risk of infection from a contaminated cannula and may develop a hematoma. There's also the risk of injury to the skin, excessive bleeding and delayed wound healing. The nurse is mainly at risk of needle pricks. Needle pricks predispose nurses to contract infections like hepatitis B and retroviral disease. Therefore, blood sampling must be done carefully and systematically.

Urine is another sample that is collected for laboratory testing. Urine is routinely collected for urinary tract infections, sexually transmitted infections and renal diseases. Proteins, blood cells, glucose and other chemicals are assayed for in the urine. A routine urine sample is collected in a container. The patient voids some urine into the container. The container is shut tightly, labeled and taken to the laboratory for testing. Urine collection can be performed as a one-time random sample or as a 24-hour collection, depending on the specific requirements of the testing.

The nurse should compare standard reference values with the samples collected from the patient. The results can either confirm or rule out a differential diagnosis.

## Potential for alteration in body systems

A nurse is expected to recognize patients with potential risks of complications and adverse disease conditions.

Due to various treatment procedures, patients have a risk of alteration in their body systems. For instance, some patients have a chance of aspiration. The entry of secretions, fluids and solids into the tracheobronchial tree is a significant risk to specific patients. Patients with nasogastric feeding tubes are at risk of aspiration of oropharyngeal or gastrointestinal secretions. Patients with an impaired gag or cough reflex find it challenging to expel contaminants in the airway, so these stray into the lungs and block the airway. Sedated patients are also at risk of aspiration.

Other patients have a risk of potential skin breakdown. Patients who are malnourished and don't eat a balanced diet have a chance of skin breakdown because the nutrients to strengthen the connective skin tissues are absent. Malnourished patients, especially in the pediatric population, have weak immune systems and are prone to infections.

Also, patients with impaired tissue perfusion and blood circulation have a potential risk of skin breakdown because not enough blood goes to the body tissues and skin and there's a higher chance of loss of skin tone.

Some other patients are predisposed to impaired or insufficient vascular perfusion. A patient who has had a traumatic injury is at risk of impaired tissue perfusion with blood. A patient who doesn't breathe well and is hyperventilating does not have enough oxygen in the blood to perfuse the tissues; hence, they are at risk of tissue hypoperfusion. This hypoperfusion can lead to shock, organ damage and even death.

Patients exposed to cigarette smoke are at risk of lung, esophageal and oral cancers. Patients with a family history of cancer are also at risk. Patients whose occupation exposes them to ultraviolet radiation are predisposed to skin cancers.

This knowledge will help the nurse identify patients at risk of various diseases quickly. After identifying these patients, it's important to educate them on how to avoid complications of their diseases and avoid developing others they are at risk for.

## Potential for complications of diagnostic tests/treatments/procedures

Invasive diagnostic tests are prone to complications. For instance, invasive procedures are prone to infections and bleeding. Also, diseases like leukemia and esophageal varices are prone to bleeding. The nurse must anticipate this and look for signs of infection or bleeding in patients.

Severe bleeding can present with features like hypotension, tachycardia, hyperventilation and abnormal breathing patterns because of acidosis in the blood. These signs and symptoms should be quickly noted, and treatment should follow immediately. The treatment focuses on restoring the fluids and blood cells lost in the blood. Transfusion of fluids like ringer's lactate and blood cells or whole blood are options.

Infections can present with a persistent fever that might be resistant to antipyretics and tepid sponging. A blood culture might be required to detect the presence of microorganisms. The patient might also be commenced on broad-spectrum antibiotics initially. Asepsis should be practiced to reduce the risk of infections in any procedure.

Proper positioning of patients is crucial in treating and preventing complications. A patient who has lost a lot of blood should be placed in a Trendelenburg position to facilitate blood flow to the brain. The head of the bed should also be elevated when the patient has a feeding tube.

### Insert, maintain or remove a nasal/oral gastrointestinal tube

Inserting a nasogastric tube begins with explaining to the patient what you're about to do, maintaining an aseptic technique and taking informed consent. The patient should be placed in a high Fowler position with nares adequately inspected. Select the best nares and measure the nasogastric from the nose to the tip of the xiphoid bone. Apply a topical/local anesthetic to the tube tip and put it into the nose. The neck should be hyperextended for proper visualization and to avoid injury to the nasopharynx. The tube should be secured with tape, a pin attaching the tube to the patient's clothes and connected to a suction tube if necessary.

Removal of the tube is quite simple. Remove the pins and tape that held the tubes in place. Ask the patient to take a deep breath and gently remove the tube. The maintenance of the nasogastric tube includes daily care. The drainage of the tube should be documented, as well as the color and contents.

**Insert, maintain or remove a peripheral intravenous line**

This is discussed earlier in the book.

**Insert, maintain and remove a urinary catheter**

A urinary catheter is used to void urine and drain the bladder. Urinary catheters come in different sizes and differ for children and adults. Insertion of a catheter is a sterile procedure that should be done aseptically.

The patient is placed in a supine position in a private room. The nurse should expose the patient's thighs and pelvic region. The patient separates the thighs to give access to the perineal area. The perineal area is covered with a sterile drape. The catheter tip is lubricated, and the urethral meatus is cleaned with an antiseptic.

The catheter is inserted into the urethral meatus and advanced above the point where urine is seen in the catheter. The nurse should inflate the catheter to secure it in the urethra. The catheter is then connected to the urine bag and attached to the patient's leg.

In maintaining the catheter, the nurse must take proper care to maintain the aseptic nature of the bag and the tubes. The urine bag should be below the abdomen and must be emptied regularly.

Removal of the catheter must be done using aseptic techniques. Most importantly, the catheter should be removed gently, disconnected from the urine bag and properly disposed of. The contents must be measured before the bag is emptied.

## Potential for complications from surgical procedures and health alterations

Nurses must acquaint themselves with the pathophysiology of various diseases and their complications.

For instance, thrombocytopenia, a decrease in the number of platelets in the blood, can be caused by various diseases. Among them are hematological diseases of the blood, such as aplastic anemia and leukemia. HIV infection is another culprit that reduces the level of platelets in the blood. Thrombocytopenia can also be a complication of using some medications. Anticonvulsants and antibiotics reduce levels of platelets. Thrombocytopenia is mostly identified when there is difficulty arresting bleeding. It can also be asymptomatic.

Wound infection is also a complication of treatment procedures like suturing and laceration repairs. Fever, malaise, tachycardia, swelling and pain are all features of infections. A nurse should be on the lookout for these signs and promptly treat them. Other complications to watch for after surgery are shock and hemorrhage.

## System Specific Assignments

A comprehensive health assessment must be performed by a nurse when seeing a patient. A focused health assessment helps to assess a specific body system.

For instance, assessing the neurological system requires assessing the cranial nerves, level of consciousness, muscle tone and mental status. A patient's level of consciousness is determined by orientation to time, place and person. Patients aren't fully conscious if they don't know the time of the day, are confused about the date or don't know where they are.

Muscle strength and tone are assessed on both the right and left of the body. Weak muscles might mean a defect in the central nervous system. They might also mean a peripheral problem. The nurse can assess the muscles and score them from 0 to 5. The muscles score zero if there's no visible contraction and score five if there's a full contraction against high resistance levels.

The 12 cranial nerves are assessed systematically. For example, the olfactory nerve is evaluated for its ability to smell. In contrast, the facial nerve is assessed for the ability to feel sensory impulses of the face and move the muscles of the face to make facial expressions.

As part of systemic-specific assignments, the glycemic level can be assessed through various signs and symptoms. Hypoglycemia commonly presents with lethargy, sweating, clumsiness, loss of consciousness, coma and even death. Conversely, hyperglycemia can present with polydipsia, urinary frequency, blurred vision, dehydration and fatigue.

**Therapeutic Procedures**

Anesthesia can be performed for therapeutic or diagnostic procedures. It prevents a client from feeling pain that would have been otherwise unbearable during a procedure. Anesthesia can be regional/local or general/systemic. Regional anesthesia is usually preferable to general anesthesia because of the side effects and risks of general anesthesia.

Regional anesthesia can be spinal anesthesia, where an anesthetic is injected into the subarachnoid space; the sites for administration are either between the L3/L4 or the L4/L5 vertebrae. Epidural anesthesia is a form of regional anesthesia where an anesthetic is injected into the epidural space above the dura mater.

General anesthesia makes the client completely unconscious. The patient is intubated and placed on mechanical ventilation throughout the procedure. The process is laborious and requires continuous monitoring. It is essential to monitor the amount of anesthetic given as it can have dangerous side effects.

Surgical procedures are sometimes the only form of therapy that can address a condition, such as tumors.

A nurse should explain each procedure's benefits, risks and side effects to the patient. Every patient has the right to reject a treatment.

A nurse must take informed consent before starting a treatment procedure.

## Physiological Adaptation

Physiological adaptation in nursing refers to the care of patients with acute, chronic or life-threatening conditions. Physiological adaptation is multidisciplinary, but nurses are at the center of the action.

### Alteration in the body system

The body has a system of checks and balances by which it regulates its functions. It also has repair mechanisms for damaged tissues and breakdown. The body can be affected by both external and internal insults. Internal insults result from internal malfunctions or disease processes. These can result in accumulated waste products, increased blood pressure and even cause electrolyte imbalances. External insults can be foreign bodies or microorganisms introduced into the body.

External insults can result in internal injury. A traumatic injury with loss of blood can lead to a lot of internal malfunctions with attendant consequences such as shock, infection, loss of consciousness and death.

The body has various mechanisms in place to take care of these alterations. However, these mechanisms can fail sometimes.

For instance, in hypertension, the heart continues to enlarge and hypertrophy occurs to compensate for the increased blood pressure. If this is not checked and corrected, hypertrophy can eventually lead to heart failure.

People have different pain thresholds. One patient might call a level of pain a 5/10 and moderate, while another calls the same level of pain a 9/10 and extreme. Both patients must be treated according to their requirements.

The presence of a robust support system is one helpful way of overcoming stress. For example, a patient in her fifties recently diagnosed with cervical cancer will need the support of her family members. Other coping mechanisms are humor, exercise and a change in perception about current disease conditions.

**Implement and monitor phototherapy**

Phototherapy treats neonatal hyperbilirubinemia and jaundice in both preterm and full-term infants. Bilirubin is a waste product produced from the breakdown of red blood cells—accumulation of excess bilirubin is deposited in the skin, eyes, brain and other internal organs.

Phototherapy uses a special type of blue light that breaks down the excess bilirubin. The light is applied directly to the infant's body. To prevent eye damage, the eyes are covered with patches and lubricating drops. This is an older method; newer methods are now available to treat neonatal jaundice.

A bilirubin blanket is a new method of treating neonatal jaundice. The complications associated with the old method of phototherapy, such as hypothermia, rashes, bronzing and retinal damage, can now be entirely avoided. The bilirubin blanket uses light with filtered-out infrared and ultraviolet light. This blanket can be used for 24 hours. It can also be used at home outside the hospital setting.

The nurse must monitor the phototherapy treatment to see if it is effective. The infant's skin color must be checked to see if the bilirubin level increases or decreases. The stool color must also be checked because the end products of bilirubin are a component of the feces. The laboratory levels of bilirubin must also be checked regularly.

## Assist with invasive procedures

Physicians and licensed practitioners do most invasive procedures, but nurses can assist them. Some invasive procedures include central venous line, needle biopsy, spinal tap and intubation.

Just like any procedure, the patient must give informed consent. The procedure must be thoroughly explained to the patient. The environment must be sterile and aseptic techniques must be employed.

For example, intubation of a patient with a mechanical ventilator begins with monitoring the vital signs like blood pressure, pulse rate and heart electrocardiogram. The suction equipment, airway supplies and intravenous supplies are then connected to the machine.

There are two types of needle biopsy—fine needle aspiration and core needle. For a needle biopsy, the patient must be positioned appropriately to expose the area of interest. The area is cleaned with an antiseptic and covered with a sterile drape. A local anesthetic is injected to numb the area for some minutes. The needle is slowly inserted and the specimen is obtained. The specimen is then sent to the laboratory for examination and the biopsy site is covered with a sterile dressing.

## Monitoring and caring for patients on a ventilator

Ventilators deliver air under pressure into the airways. The air under pressure keeps the alveoli open so there can be gaseous exchange in the blood that flows through the alveoli. Ventilators increase the oxygen saturation of a patient and lung capacity and decrease the breathing workload on the patient.

Nurses must be aware of the complications of using ventilators. For instance, the alveoli can over-distend due to increased air pressure from the ventilator. This overdistension can lead to pneumothorax and increased work of breathing in the patient.

Oxygen toxicity is another complication. There is a tendency for the blood to be oversaturated with oxygen. Regular monitoring of the oxygen saturation level and level of carbon dioxide on the arterial blood gas machine is a way of preventing oxygen toxicity.

Infections are another possibility. Bacteria and microbes can hide in the inner lining of ventilator tubes and cause infections in patients. Pneumonia is a common disease acquired by patients on ventilators. Basic aseptic techniques like handwashing can prevent the transfer of bacteria to patients.

**Perform Suctioning**

The airways, including the nose, nasopharyngeal, tracheal airways and other artificial airways, must always be kept patent. Suctioning is the mechanical aspiration of pulmonary secretions from the airways.

Oxygen is administered before suctioning to maintain the airways during suctioning. A sterile glove is worn, and the tip of the suction catheter is lubricated. The catheter is slowly advanced into the patient's airways to remove secretions. This process can be repeated until the airways are clear.

**Perform wound care and dressing change**

Wounds can be open or closed. Closed wounds are usually due to blunt trauma and can result in internal bleeding and closed fractures. Wounds usually require some level of dressing and care. Open wounds can be abrasions, punctures, lacerations, gunshot wounds or surgical wounds.

Wound care and dressing change is an aseptic procedure. The wound is cleaned first with normal saline and other antiseptic solutions like methylated spirits or povidone-iodine. The wound is cleaned from inside to outside, from the less contaminated area to the most contaminated area. Gauze is used to remove any debris and pus.

The wound area is inspected regularly. The color, size, presence of pus, surrounding structures and odor of the pus are examined. The drainages of the wound can be bloody, serous, serosanguinous and purulent. After cleaning, a new gauze or bandage plaster is used to dress the wound.

The frequency of dressing depends on factors like the nature of the wound, the location, how much discharge is being produced, if it is infected or not and the preference of the physician.

**Perform postoperative care**

Postoperative care is given to a patient after a surgical procedure. It is a critical part of the recovery process of any patient.

The patient is monitored after surgery by the nurse. The vital signs are first examined. The pulse rate and blood pressure are measured. The respiratory system is also examined. Patients just recovering from general anesthesia in surgery are at risk of dysphagia and laryngospasms. They might also feel some lightheadedness and drowsiness, which will eventually wear off. So the patients should be reassured.

Patients that have had spinal or epidural anesthesia should not raise their heads for a few hours after the procedure to prevent postdural puncture headaches.

The nurse must always ensure that the postoperative order is adequately documented and followed. Any clarifications should be made before care is commenced.

A patient with a cast must be monitored for pain and limb alignment. The patient's limb pulses and vital signs need to be adequately monitored.

**Provide pulmonary hygiene**

Pulmonary hygiene consists of techniques to clear the airways. The airway structures should be patent at all times so that air can flow in and out freely. Simple hygiene techniques include coughing, deep breathing and postural drainage. Advanced techniques include percussion and vibrations.

Coughing and deep breathing are simple techniques that can be done by asking the patient to take a deep breath through the nose and exhale through the mouth. This is done three times, followed by coughing. This process can be repeated as much as possible to clear the airways.

Postural drainage means placing the patient in different positions until respiratory secretions are completely drained. For example, the patient rests flat and the bed is elevated to a 45-degree position. This drains respiratory secretions from the posterior bronchus. The patient can lay supine with the head of the bed elevated to 45 degrees to drain the anterior apical segment of the upper lobes of the lungs.

Percussion is an advanced technique that involves placing a hand over an area of the lung and gently tapping on that area for about a minute while the patient breathes in to hyperinflate the lungs. The patient is prone and the bed is elevated to a 45-degree position. Percussion is usually done with postural drainage.

Postural drainage is very useful in patients with conditions that produce excessive secretions, such as COPD or bronchiectasis.

**Provide ostomy care and education**

Ostomies are surgical operations that can be done to divert the bowels (colostomy). Tracheal ostomies can also be performed. Ostomy care and education involves informing the patient about the ostomy, its purpose, the risks of the surgery and care after the surgery. All these responsibilities lie in the hands of a nurse.

The surgical wound site is examined as part of care for ostomies. Nurses maintain the tubes' patency and change them as necessary. For tracheostomies, the nurse monitors the respiratory secretions input and output. The nurse must ensure the tubes are patent and changed at the right time.

Other routine care should not be neglected while taking care of the surgery site. These include vital signs monitoring and fluid input/output.

**Manage the care of clients receiving peritoneal dialysis**

Dialysis replaces the function of the kidneys. This machine clears waste products from the body and balances the pH of the blood. As a result of kidney failure, waste products accumulate in the body, which is dangerous to the patient. There are two types of dialysis: hemodialysis and peritoneal dialysis.

Hemodialysis is a form of dialysis via an AV fistula or a central vascular line. This process can take three to five hours. The AV graft is placed into the patient's upper arm. The AV graft is preferred to the vascular access line because it stays longer and lowers the risk of infection. An arteriovenous fistula (AV) is a connection between an artery and vein done three months before the dialysis to allow for maturity. During this process, the nurse monitors the input and output of the patient. The nurse can administer any ordered anticoagulants during this process. The patient's vitals are recorded, including blood pressure, pulse rate and oxygen saturation.

Peritoneal dialysis is done by passing a catheter into the peritoneal space. This option is for patients who are at risk of complications from medications given on hemodialysis. Patients with poor venous access can get peritoneal dialysis. Nurses measure and monitor the input and output of the patient. The color of the fluid drained out of the patient is also recorded. Nurses also monitor for complications of dialysis treatment— for example, peritonitis and infections from the tubes harboring bacteria.

<u>**Fluid and Electrolyte Balance**</u>

Fluids and electrolytes are significant components of the internal milieu. Electrolytes are responsible for maintaining the balance between the extracellular and intracellular compartments. Fluids are responsible for the functioning of the heart muscles and major organs of the body. These electrolytes must be monitored regularly.

**Identify signs and symptoms of client fluid and/or electrolyte imbalance**

Some significant electrolytes in the body include sodium, potassium, calcium, magnesium and chloride.

**Potassium**

Potassium is the most abundant intracellular electrolyte. Potassium is primarily responsible for muscle contractions and the normal functioning of the nervous system. Potassium can be high or low in the body, indicating hyperkalemia or hypokalemia.

Hyperkalemia is an elevation of the potassium levels in the blood above the expected standard value. Features of hyperkalemia include muscle paralysis, generalized body weakness, nausea and cardiac arrhythmias. These signs are not exclusive to hyperkalemia, but hyperkalemia must be at the top of the list of possible causes. Hyperkalemia can be treated with dialysis and potassium-lowering drugs.

Hypokalemia is the reduction in the potassium labels in the blood below the usual standard. Hypokalemia can be a result of diarrhea, vomiting and diaphoresis. Hypokalemia is characterized by muscle weakness, tingling, numbness, constipation and even cardiac arrest. Treatment is supplemental potassium.

**Sodium**

Sodium is responsible for the fluid balance between the extracellular and intracellular compartments of the body. Sodium also keeps the nervous system active and helps in muscle contractions. Sodium levels can be high or low in the plasma.

Hypernatremia is an elevation of the body's sodium level. Hypernatremia can arise from several illnesses and conditions like diabetes insipidus, diarrhea, vomiting and Cushing's syndrome. Features of hypernatremia include thirst, agitation, restlessness and confusion. Identifying the underlying cause of hypernatremia and limiting dietary intake of sodium is critical to treating the condition.

Hyponatremia is a reduction in the sodium level in the body below the usual standard. Thyroid gland diseases, renal failure and diuretic medications can cause hyponatremia. The condition is characterized by confusion, vomiting, nausea, headaches and muscle weakness. Hyponatremia is treated by identifying the underlying conditions causing the hyponatremia. Fluid restriction and intravenous sodium are other options for treating hyponatremia.

**Fluid Imbalances**

Hypervolemia is an increase in fluid in the blood. This increases the blood volume and may increase the electrolytes in the blood. Hypervolemia is caused by increased sodium and fluid overload from the intravenous fluid infusion. The clinical features of hypervolemia are hypertension, dyspnea, shortness of breath and peripheral edema in the feet and hands. Treatment includes sodium and fluid restrictions and treating any underlying conditions causing hypervolemia.

Hypovolemia is a reduction in the fluid in the blood. Hypovolemia may occur as a result of bleeding, vomiting and diarrhea. This deficit in fluids in the blood can lead to shock, reduced cardiac output, coma and even death. Resuscitation is the first line of treatment. Infusion of intravenous fluids like ringers' lactate can expand the blood volume.

## Hemodynamics

Hemodynamics is the study of how blood flows through the blood vessels. It studies the factors responsible for free flow. It also studies the turbulent flow of blood in blood vessels.

**Monitor and maintain arterial lines**

Arterial lines can be placed in various arteries like the femoral, brachial and radial arteries. These lines are inserted via a surgical procedure to monitor the patient's blood pressure. Arterial lines can also be used to obtain frequent blood samples. Nurses should know the complications, like infections, trauma, hematomas and scar tissue formation.

Arterial lines are used for patients with atherosclerosis, clotting disorders and impaired circulation. Nurses monitor the hemodynamic status of patients with arterial lines. They also anticipate complications and manage them accordingly.

**Manage the care of patients with telemetry**

Telemetry is the continuous monitoring and recording of ECG strips. It is mostly done by a telemetry technician, but nurses can also monitor telemetry. When there is a problem with the patient's ECG, the nurse has to interpret the ECG and decide on the next course of action.

**Manage the care of a patient with a pacing device**

The care of a patient with a pacing device begins with educating the patient about the reason for the pacemaker. The nurse should be aware of the complication of having a pacemaker. Complications of having a pacing device include pneumothorax, hemothorax, perforation of the pacemaker lead and cardiac tamponade.

These complications are identified by shortness of breath, chest pain and low blood pressure. The nurse monitors the ECG for the failure of the pacemaker. The insertion site of the pacemaker should be assessed for bleeding and infections. The nurse should maintain bed rest and avoid giving the patient heparin or aspirin.

**Illness Management**

Illness management begins with educating the patient about acute and chronic conditions. The education of patients includes information about the pathophysiology of the disease condition. The nurse should be able to explain how the disease process began. The patient should be told about the risk factors predisposing to the diseases. The signs and symptoms of the disease should be explained to the patient so they can be reported to the doctor if present.

Treatable signs and symptoms of chronic diseases should be explained to the patient. The patient should also be told about the treatment procedures and the financial cost of each treatment. Nurses should teach patients about home care strategies for their illnesses. Patients should receive the follow-up schedule as part of the treatment plan.

Patients with impaired ventilation/oxygenation should be assessed with pulmonary function tests like pulse oximetry, spirometry, lung compliance and forced vital capacity. Nurses should manage these patients by regularly monitoring the results of these tests.

## Test 1 Questions

(1) The term "advance directives" refers to _____.

(A) Documents given in advance of a medical condition

(B) Documents given when the patient is in a coma

(C) Legal documentation on how a patient should be handled at all times

(D) Legal documentation on how clients should be handled if they are unable to communicate

(2) What is the responsibility of a nurse when a patient has already prepared advance directives?

(A) Document them in patient records.

(B) Inform other health care personnel that need to know.

(C) Ensure they are carried out if the occasion arises.

(D) All of the above.

(3) What types of tasks can be delegated?

(A) Set routines

(B) Tasks that require lower levels of professional judgment

(C) Needs of clients in stable condition

(D) Tasks that require higher levels of quick judgment calls


(4) What are the five rights of delegation?

(A) Person, task, perception, circumstance, supervision

(B) Person, task, circumstance, direction, supervision

(C) Person, task, skill, direction, supervision

(D) Person, task, equipment, remuneration, supervision


(5) What type of health care reimbursement system involves health care facilities receiving payments for the care they render based on the cost?

(A) Prospective reimbursement

(B) Retrogressive reimbursement

(C) Progressive reimbursement

(D) Retrospective reimbursement

(6) What key feature must be considered when developing health care plans for clients?

(A) Individualization

(B) Movement

(C) Evaluation /

(D) All of the above

(7) One of your junior nursing staff members refused to allow a client to look through his medical records. What should you do as an RN?

(A) Apologize to the client and allow him to view his records,

(B) Support your staff.

(C) Educate your staff on HIPAA. /

(D) All of the above.

*Health Insurance Protability act and accountability act*

(8) According to the Bill of Rights, patients can choose _____.

(A) Their health care provider

(B) The type of health care plans that they do not want

(C) The type of health care plans that they want

(D) All of the above

(9) Advocacy does not include _____.

(A) Updating other nursing staff about client advocacy

(B) Documenting the needs of the client

(C) Communicating the needs of clients orally to other nursing staff

(D) Playing multiple roles for effectiveness

(10) A patient presents with pentazocine addiction. The nurse decides to call in a psychologist, psychotherapist and physician. What has the nurse demonstrated?

(A) Crisis intervention

(B) Recognition of appropriate resources for referral needs

(C) Client assessment

(D) B and C

(11) What is the right order of resuscitation?

(A) Airway, breathing, circulation

(B) Breathing, airway, circulation

(C) Circulation, breathing, airway

(D) Circulation, airway, breathing

ABC
CAB

178

(12) What is a blameless environment?

(A) One without fault

(B) One where mistakes are not readily made

(C) One where mistakes are seen as opportunities for improvement

(D) One where there is a focus on the individual who made the error

(13) Values like the population of clients on the ward can be evaluated with _____.

(A) Core measures

(B) Outcome measures

(C) Quality measures

(D) Quantity measures

(14) Which of the following steps is not common to all performance improvement methods?

(A) Problem definition

(B) Root cause analysis

(C) Narrowing down

(D) None of the above

(15) Which health care personnel can manage an unstable case effectively?

(A) LPNs

(B) RNs

(C) Nursing assistants

(D) All of the above

(16) In cases of child abuse, which health care personnel must be involved?

(A) Physical therapists

(B) Occupational therapists

(C) Nutritionists

(D) Social workers

(17) At what point do people provide logical or illogical reasons for what brought them to the point of conflict?

(A) Frustration

(B) Anger

(C) Conceptualization

(D) Action


(18) Unhealthy methods of conflict resolution include _____.

(A) Avoidance, competition, mediation

(B) Mediation, compromise, collaboration

(C) Avoidance, accommodating without addressing issues, competition

(D) None of the above

(19) A nurse working in the emergency room has a very busy afternoon. She has four patients that need attention: a teenager with an adverse reaction (fever and shivering) from an ongoing blood transfusion; a middle-aged man with pain from osteoarthritis in his right knee; a 25-year-old man involved in an auto crash who has lost a lot of blood and an elderly woman in for her weekly chemotherapy. In what order should the nurse attend to the patients?

(A) Teenager, middle-aged man, elderly woman, young man

(B) Middle-aged man, elderly woman, young man, teenager

(C) Young man, middle-aged man, teenager, elderly woman

(D) Teenager, young man, middle-aged man, elderly woman

(20) Which of the following should not determine priorities?

(A) Pathophysiology

(B) Acuity

(C) Race

(D) All of the above

(21) How is the effectiveness of care determined?

(A) Cost of care

(B) Acuity of care

(C) Recovery of client

(D) Disease follows pathophysiology


(22) What is one main feature of ethical dilemmas?

(A) Ethical standards conflict with nurse's beliefs.

(B) Ethical standards conflict with client interests.

(C) Client interests align with ethical standards.

(D) Clients have no say in ethical dilemmas.


(23) What is the purpose of evaluation in nursing practice?

(A) It helps nurses to better commit to their responsibilities.

(B) It involves witch hunting.

(C) It favors only those at the top.

(D) None of the above.

(24) What is the right way to input information for clients?

(A) 08/12/20 1020 hrs. IM Diclofenac 75 mg stat given. Pain has subsided.

(B) 08/12/20 1020 hrs. IM Diclofenac 75 mg total dose given. Pain reported 2/10.

(C) 08/12/20 1020 hrs IV Diclofenac 75 mg given. Patient is feeling better.

(D) 09/10/20 1145 hrs IM Diclofenac 75 mg STAT given. Patient reports pain as 2/10.

STAT → urgent / immediate

(25) Your friend's brother, Joe, calls you asking for information about one of his friends on your ward who was involved in an accident. He is aware there is a fracture but wants to know if any of his friend's organs were affected. What is your most appropriate response?

(A) "It was just his right leg."

(B) "Joe, please get off my phone. Never ask me about client issues."

(C) "I am sorry, Joe. I can't give you that information."

(D) "Please ask your friend if he wants me to tell you."

(26) How can you communicate with a blind patient?

(A) Signs

(B) Verbally

(C) Braille → dot. projection for blind people to read.

(D) B and C


(27) The physician on call the previous shift forgot to document a medication to be given at 0700 hrs. He calls to ask you to give it. What do you say?

(A) "I cannot give the medication because you did not document it."

(B) "I cannot give the medication because you did not document it. I suggest you ask another physician to come document it."

(C) "Please don't tell me to do this again; it is against the law."

(D) "I cannot give the medication because you did not document it. Verbal orders are recognized only during emergencies. I suggest you ask another physician to come document it."

(28) When is target screening performed?

(A) When a patient is undergoing a routine check-up

(B) When a client is at risk of a certain disease

(C) To rule out a possible condition in a patient

(D) B and C

(29) Health history does not _____.

(A) Involve open-ended questions

(B) Involve closed-ended questions

(C) Involve interview-style questions

(D) Help clients express themselves more

(30) How can a nurse help a client who has unprotected sex regularly with multiple sexual partners?

(A) Counsel on abstinence

(B) Counsel on the use of condoms

(C) Counsel on avoiding multiple sexual partners

(D) All of the above

(31) How can a nurse help prevent malnutrition among children in a client's family?

(A) Educate the parents about a balanced diet.

(B) Educate the children about a balanced diet.

(C) Counsel the parents on cooking techniques.

(D) Counsel the parents on finances.


(32) Mr. Alex has always believed that he can control his fate. He has been diagnosed with cancer but still believes he must do all he can to live healthily. Mr. Alex can be said to have _____.

(A) Internal locus

(B) External locus

(C) Experiential readiness

(D) Mental readiness

(33) How do nurses assess a client's knowledge of health-promoting behaviors?

D

(A) Observation

(B) Formal and informal questions

(C) Questionnaires

(D) All of the above


(34) What age group coincides with Piaget's sensorimotor stage?

*tault by family nurse*

(A) Neonates

(B) Infants

(C) Toddlers

(D) Preschoolers

(35) A mother complains about her six-year-old, who has begun to challenge her authority at home. After reassuring her that this comes with age, what should the nurse counsel her to help her child avoid?

D

(A) Smoking

(B) Unsupervised swimming

(C) Falls

(D) All of the above


(36) What are some of the concerns of Erikson's generativity vs. stagnation stage?

(A) / ℞

(A) Care of children and aging parents

(B) Seeking purpose

(C) Self-consciousness

(D) Retirement

(37) What is the significance of decreased hepatic and renal function in the elderly?

B

(A) Avoiding falls

(B) Prescription medications

(C) Isolation from family

(D) All of the above

(38) What is the most accurate method of determining EDD?

(A) LMP

(B) Ultrasound

(C) Ovulation date

(D) None of the above

There is no answer

(39) A woman presents to the hospital in the second stage of labor. What should a nurse expect at this stage?

(A) Braxton-Hicks contraction

(B) 2 cm cervical dilatation

(C) Delivery of the fetus

(D) 6 cm cervical dilatation

(40) What should be used to clean the umbilical cord?

(A) Alcohol

(B) Normal saline

(C) Warm water

(D) All of the above

(41) Which of the following could be a potential sign of an allergic reaction?

(A) Difficulty breathing

(B) Hypotension

(C) Tingling sensation

(D) All of the above

191

(42) What is the right thing to do in the event of an allergic reaction?

(A) Send the patient home since available treatment options are not compatible.

(B) Document the client's allergic reaction for future purposes.

(C) Move the client to another room to stop the allergic reaction.

(D) Contact the CDC.

(43) Which category of patient would be more prone to a fall?

(A) A mentally unstable, restrained patient

(B) A 30-year-old sedated and unrestrained patient

(C) An 83-year-old patient in a room with low-glare floors

(D) A day-old baby in the ICU

(44) Most state laws require infants and toddlers to be strapped in car seats until

_____.

(A) They are 12 years old.

(B) They are 4'9" in height.

(C) They weigh 80 pounds.

(D) They are 4'9" or 80 pounds. D *possible*

(45) Which of the following precautionary measures should be implemented for patients at risk of seizures?

(A) Padding and raising the client's bed for better positioning and comfortability

(B) Having oxygen and suction equipment on standby at all times

(C) Putting the client in a private room to promote client confidentiality and avoid embarrassment

(D) All of the above

(46) What is not the right procedure to take to identify clients properly?

(A) Staying mindful of clients who might be at a higher risk of identification errors

(B) Using identifiers like clients' date of birth and codes

(C) Using one distinct identifier alongside the room number of clients for easy and efficient identification

(D) Adding extra identifiers in the event of more than one client who has the same name


(47) Does the RN have a right to question treatment orders that seem out of place?

(A) No.

(B) Yes.

(C) It depends on who made the prescription.

(D) It is subject to each health care facility's rules.

(48) Which of the following is incorrect about code names used in emergencies and disasters?

(A) Code Gray is the appropriate code for communicating infant abduction.

(B) Code Red and Code Orange are used for fire hazards and chemical spills respectively.

(C) Code Blue is popular for communicating the occurrence of a cardiac arrest.

(D) Code Brown is the code used for indicating a severe weather disaster.


(49) What is the right action to take when managing clients and using common hospital equipment and facilities?

(A) Using the muscles of the back when lifting an object to ensure a strong and sturdy grip

(B) Facing the person or object you are about to lift while keeping your feet close together to provide a secure base

(C) None of the above

(D) All of the above

(50) Before assigning assistive devices to clients, RNs should consider various factors to determine clients' ability to use the devices. These factors include but are not limited to _____.

(A) The distance of the client's home to the health care facility and the weight of the client

(B) The cognitive ability of the client and the person's religious or cultural affiliations

(C) The client's income level and muscular strength

(D) The developmental stage of the client and the environment


(51) What is not a general principle for handling biohazardous waste?

(A) Avoid reusing materials designed for single use.

(B) Properly clean and disinfect non-single-use materials.

(C) Rigorously wash your hands before handling any biohazardous material.

(D) Dispose of biohazardous material in any trash can available.

(52) What should nurses look out for when inspecting equipment?

(A) Loose or missing equipment parts

(B) Frayed electrical cords

(C) Overloaded power outlets

(D) All of the above


(53) What should nurses do to prepare for security threats?

(A) Delegate security responsibilities to other staff members.

(B) Review policies and procedures only in the event of a security breach.

(C) Participate in periodic training and mock drills.

(D) Hire security experts who will manage situations when they arise.


(54) What are the modes of transmission of pathogens?

(A) Airborne, contact, droplet and vector-borne

(B) Airborne, droplet, direct and indirect

(C) Vector-borne, direct, indirect and airborne

(D) Contact, vector-borne, direct and indirect

(55) What is an example of a vector-borne transmission mode?

(A) Touching a contaminated surface and then touching one's mouth

(B) Inhaling respiratory droplets from a person infected with a contagious disease

(C) Getting bitten by a mosquito carrying the West Nile virus

(D) Shaking hands with a person who has a cold


(56) When should handwashing be done?

(A) Before contact with a client

(B) When the hands have been soiled

(C) After touching equipment, instruments and other treatment materials with bare hands

(D) All of the above

(57) What are aseptic techniques?

(A) Measures taken to prevent the transfer of disease-causing organisms from one person or object to the other

(B) Measures taken to render microorganisms ineffective for causing infections

(C) Precautionary measures used for all clients to prevent the spread of infection

(D) Measures taken to prevent the spread of specific infections


(58) What is the appropriate procedure for reporting and communicating infectious diseases?

(A) Reports should go to the client's family members.

(B) Reports should go to the Centers for Disease Control and Prevention.

(C) Reports should go to the local hospital.

(D) Reports should go to the nurse's supervisor.

(59) Which of the following is the responsibility of RNs concerning infection control and prevention measures?

(A) Test clients for infection before they're admitted.

(B) Ensure that staff members adhere to infection control measures.

(C) Plan and evaluate educational activities on safety for clients.

(D) Administer antibiotics to infected patients.


(60) What should be considered when selecting an appropriate restraint for a client?

(A) The patient's level of consciousness

(B) The patient's mobility

(C) The patient's age

(D) The patient's preference

(61) Vital signs include all of the following except _____.

(A) Blood pressure

(B) Respiratory rate

(C) Pulse rate

(D) BMI

(62) What sounds are heard while checking for blood pressure?

(A) Korotkoff sounds

(B) Waltz sounds

(C) Lead sounds

(D) Schmitz sounds

(63) What is the first step before performing any test?

(A) Confirm the doctor's order.

(B) Identify the patient.

(C) Prepare the materials.

(D) A and B.

(64) What does the ECG machine record?

(A) Electrical impulses of the heart

(B) Sinus waves

(C) Mechanical impulses of the heart

(D) Potential energy of the heart

(65) What is not a method for blood sample collection?

(A) Arterial sampling

(B) Venipuncture

(C) Finger prick

(D) None of the above

(66) The most important risk to the nurse during a venipuncture is _____.

(A) Injury to the skin

(B) Excessive bleeding

(C) Delayed wound healing

(D) Needle prick

(67) How would a nurse prevent hematoma formation while taking samples?

(A) Ask the patient to flex the elbow after sample collection.

(B) Apply pressure on the sample collection site.

(C) Ensure the sample is only taken once.

(D) Remove the tourniquet as fast as possible.


(68) Which of the following patients have the least risk of aspiration?

(A) Patient with NG tubes

(B) Patients with impaired gag reflex

(C) Sedated patients

(D) Conscious patients


(69) What is the greatest immediate concern for a patient who has lost a lot of blood from a traumatic injury?

(A) Hypovolemic shock

(B) Neurogenic shock

(C) Hypothermia

(D) Infection

(70) Malnourishment can lead to _____.

(A) Infections

(B) Weak immune system

(C) Skin breakdown

(D) All of the above

(71) A patient presenting with a persistent fever that is resistant to antipyretics might urgently need all of the following except a/an _____.

(A) CBC

(B) Blood culture

(C) EUCR

(D) CT scan

(72) What factors should be noted before removing a nasogastric tube?

(A) Drainage quantity

(B) Color

(C) Content

(D) All of the above

(73) Where is the tourniquet placed when securing IV access?

(A) Below the selected site

(B) At the selected site

(C) A few inches above the selected site

(D) None of the above


(74) The catheter enters the bladder by passing through the _____.

(A) Urethral meatus

(B) Urethra

(C) A and B

(D) None of the above


(75) Which cranial nerve is involved in smell?

(A) Ophthalmic nerve

(B) Olfactory nerve

(C) Trigeminal nerve

(D) Optic nerve

(76) Symptoms of hypoglycemia include all of the following except _____.

(A) Lethargy

(B) Sweating

(C) Polydipsia

(D) Clumsiness

(77) Types of anesthesia include _____.

(A) Regional, general

(B) Full, partial

(C) Strong, weak

(D) Upper limb block, lower limb block

(78) What kind of anesthesia is given above the dura mater?

(A) Spinal

(B) Epidural

(C) Bier's block

(D) General anesthesia

(79) What type of insult is a gunshot injury?

(A) External

(B) Internal

(C) Internal and external

(D) None of the above

(80) Bilirubin is formed from the _____.

(A) Breakdown of fats

(B) Breakdown of RBCs

(C) Formation of RBCs

(D) Breakdown of hepatocytes

(81) Initial steps to performing an invasive procedure include _____.

(A) Gathering materials

(B) Obtaining informed consent

(C) Explaining the procedure to the patient

(D) All of the above

(82) Why are ventilators used?

(A) To increase the breathing workload of the patient

(B) To reduce the breathing workload on the patient

(C) For procedures requiring local anesthesia

(D) For procedures requiring conscious sedation

(83) What is suctioning?

(A) Natural aspiration of pulmonary secretions

(B) Artificial use of air to prevent the collapse of the lungs

(C) Artificial aspiration of pulmonary secretions

(D) Preoxygenation of the patient before surgery

(84) Wound dressing materials do not include _____.

(A) Povidone

(B) Methylated spirit

(C) Honey

(D) None of the above

(85) What are the first steps to perform once a patient is received from surgery?

(A) Examine vital signs.

(B) Check the surgery site.

(C) Request postoperative orders.

(D) Request handover notes.

(86) Simple techniques for pulmonary hygiene include _____.

(A) Coughing, deep breathing, vibrations

(B) Deep breathing, vibrations and percussion

(C) Vibrations and percussion

(D) Coughing and postural drainage

(87) Ostomies are surgical operations done to create _____.

(A) Heart chambers

(B) Openings from the outside to the inside

(C) Organs

(D) Openings from the inside to the outside

(88) One complication of peritoneal dialysis that a nurse must look out for in patients is _____.

(A) Peritonitis

(B) Headaches

(C) Vomiting

(D) Swollen lower limbs


(89) What is the position of the AV graft used in dialysis?

(A) Upper limb

(B) Lower thigh

(C) Chest

(D) Elbow


(90) Which of the following is not an electrolyte in the body?

(A) Sodium

(B) Magnesium

(C) Calcium

(D) Mercury

(91) A patient is observed to experience cardiac arrhythmias. What investigation should be ordered immediately and why?

(A) CBC, infection

(B) Blood culture, infection

(C) Peripheral blood film, leukemia

(D) EUCR, hyperkalemia


(92) What is a common cause of hyponatremia?

(A) Diuretics

(B) Dialysis

(C) Vomiting

(D) Headaches

(93) What is a complication of hypovolemia that can lead to death quickly if not addressed in time?

(A) Vomiting

(B) Hypothermia

(C) Shock

(D) All of the above


(94) Examples of blood volume expanders are _____.

(A) 50% dextrose water

(B) 50% dextrose saline

(C) Ringer's lactate

(D) Mannitol


(95) What is telemetry?

(A) Continuous monitoring of an EEG

(B) Continuous monitoring and recording of an ECG

(C) One-time measurement and recording of an ECG

(D) None of the above

(96) How does a patient present when there is hemothorax?

(A) Shortness of breath

(B) Low blood pressure

(C) Chest might not rise fully on the affected side

(D) A and C

(97) Arterial lines can be used to _____.

(A) Monitor the patient's blood pressure

(B) Obtain frequent blood samples

(C) A and B

(D) None of the above

(98) Examples of pulmonary function tests include _____.

(A) Spirometry

(B) Blood glucose

(C) Chest X-rays

(D) Chest CT scans

(99) How do nurses help a patient manage a disease at home?

(A) Teach the client to come in when there is any sign.

(B) Teach the client home care strategies for the illness.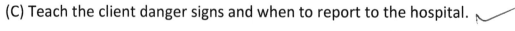

(C) Teach the client danger signs and when to report to the hospital.

(D) B and C.


(100) An 80-year-old woman is a known patient with diabetes mellitus and has been in treatment for over 30 years. She is admitted for a routine check-up. Which of the following basic assessments is most important in this patient?

(A) Mobility assessment

(B) Hearing assessment

(C) Speech assessment

(D) Visual assessment

(101) A 65-year-old man was admitted to the ER with a complaint of inability to pass stool for the past week. Previous digital rectal examination findings revealed a full rectum with hardened stool. As the nurse on duty, what is your most likely assessment?

(A) Constipation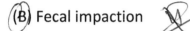

(B) Fecal impaction

(C) Intestinal obstruction

(D) Volvulus

(102) During a mobility assessment of a patient admitted for thoracic spine transection, which of these statements is true?

(A) Mobility issues are acquired from predisposing factors.

(B) Muscle contraction as a parameter for mobility assessment is scored on a scale of 0 to 6.

(C) Mobility issues can affect other systems aside from the musculoskeletal system.

(D) Mobility issues are usually unifactorial.

(103) A 50-year-old woman being managed for advanced breast cancer complains of pain. Which of the following is true about pain management and evaluation?

(A) Acute pain is usually described based on the severity of the pain.

(B) Pharmacological treatment is always indicated in pain management.

(C) Pain is usually a complication of treatment in oncology cases. X

(D) Nonpharmacological comfort interventions can be effective in the management of pain. ✓


(104) A patient was managed for major depression and was placed on amitriptyline and lorazepam. The patient is complaining of excessive somnolence. What is the next best course of action?

(A) Increase the dosage of medication.

(B) Stop medication immediately.

(C) Document for possible revision of medications and reduction of dosage.

(D) Dissuade the patient's fears and continue the current medication at the  present dosage.

(105) An unconscious patient was admitted following RTA with a cervical and thoracic spine fracture. What is the most appropriate method to prevent bed sores in this patient?

(A) Regular turning in bed

(B) Use of a waterbed

(C) Adequate rehydration

(D) Regular application of zinc oxide cream


(106) A patient who injected a toxic substance that is primarily eliminated by the kidneys is brought to the ER. Which of the following methods is ineffective in enhancing renal elimination?

(A) Increase intravenous fluid intake

(B) Administration of diuretics

(C) Ensured adequate blood flow and perfusion

(D) Suprapubic (bladder) massage

(107) A patient was admitted and managed for constipation. What is not an appropriate part of the evaluation and care of the patient?

(A) Increasing intravenous fluid intake

(B) Assessment of dietary intake

(C) Assessment of bowel habits

(D) Possible enema if indicated

(108) A 12-year-old child who is being managed for sepsis is noticed to be running a fever with a temperature of 39.1 °C. What is not an appropriate line of care?

(A) Administration of antipyretics

(B) Exposing the child adequately and tepid sponging

(C) Increasing fluid intake

(D) Encouraging ambulation

(109) A patient is being treated for traumatic brain injury following a road traffic accident. The patient is observed to be confused. What is an inappropriate line of care for this patient?

(A) Sedate the patient.

(B) Ensure the bed railings are up.

(C) Lightly restrain the patient in bed.

(D) Adequately counsel the relatives.


(110) A 35-year-old woman is being evaluated for cholecystitis. She is found to be morbidly obese and has been previously diagnosed with binge eating. Which counsel is inappropriate?

(A) Avoidance/reduction of fatty meal intake and fast foods

(B) Weight reduction

(C) Frequent small meals

(D) Regular fasting

(111) An unconscious patient is being managed in the intensive care unit by the nurse on duty. What is the inappropriate way to feed this patient?

(A) Commence total parenteral nutrition where available.

(B) Spoon-feed the patient while propped up in bed.

(C) Ensure glucose-containing intravenous fluids are given.

(D) Pass an orogastric tube to feed with a blended diet.


(112) A seven-month-old infant is brought to the pediatric outpatient clinic on account of poor weight gain following weaning off breast milk. What is an inappropriate question to ask when evaluating this patient?

(A) Weaning diet

(B) History of maternal illness in pregnancy

(C) Birth and current weight of the child

(D) Appetite and dietary habit

(113) A 68-year-old woman has left hip hemiarthroplasty for an acetabular fracture. Which mobility assistive device is best to use with this patient?

(A) Zimmer's walking frame

(B) Elbow crutches

(C) Walking cane

(D) Wheelchair


(114) Which of the following is not true about substance abuse?

(A) It is the overuse of addictive substances.

(B) It is the use of unprescribed substances.

(C) It can lead to physical dependence.

(D) It cannot happen without dependence.

(115) Matt has been smoking for 17 years. His doctor has confirmed some lung changes that are looking carcinogenic, but Matt still keeps smoking. What is the term for this?

(A) Dependence

(B) Addiction

(C) Withdrawal symptoms

(D) Substance abuse


(116) A patient presents to the ER complaining of an inability to sleep. On examination, you find he has needle marks on his upper limbs. He is also moving slowly and has remarkably poor hygiene. What should be your next steps?

(A) Call the police.

(B) Evaluate the patient using CAGE-AID.

(C) Refer the patient.

(D) Prescribe medications for his symptoms.

(117) Tools to assess client support systems include _____.

(A) Interval follow-up evaluation, range of impaired functioning

(B) CAGE-AID, drug abuse screening test

(C) MAS test, CAGE-AID

(D) All of the above

(118) When there is a massive earthquake, thousands of people are displaced and lives are lost. What type of crisis is this?

(A) Situational

(B) Developmental

(C) Adventitious

(D) None of the above

(119) Which is not a component of Leininger's transcultural nursing theory?

(A) Cultural interference and restructuring

(B) Cultural preservation and maintenance

(C) Cultural care negation and accommodation

(D) Cultural care repatterning and restructuring

(120) A patient diagnosed with stage IV breast cancer has been unable to eat since she received the news. She used to be lively but has now become very depressed. Her family members are concerned. You notice she is looking dehydrated and weak. What can you do to help?

(A) Set up infusions.

(B) Refer the patient to a psychologist.

(C) Counsel the relatives.

(D) All of the above.

(121) Examples of biological needs that impact family functioning include _____.

(A) Ill health

(B) Disability

(C) Unemployment

(D) A and B

(122) Chris lost his father two days ago, but he has repeatedly been asking him to come back. He says that his dad just took one of his long evening walks and will soon come back home. What stage of the Kübler-Ross model is this?

(A) Denial

(B) Depression

(C) Bargaining

(D) Acceptance


(123) Schizophrenia belongs to what class of mental illnesses?

(A) Psychotic disorder

(B) Personality mental disorders cluster C

(C) Personality mental disorders cluster A

(D) Personality mental disorder cluster B

(124) A woman presents with a very low PCV. On taking her history, you find she does not believe in or want a blood transfusion. What is your next course of action?

(A) Try to convince her.

(B) Document her stance and seek alternatives.

(C) Explain the risks associated with her decision.

(D) B and C.


(125) At what stage of Hans Selye's theory do physiological responses show an upset in the body's homeostasis?

(A) Alarm

(B) Resistance

(C) Exhaustion

(D) All of the above

(126) Which of the following should be avoided when communicating with a patient?

(A) Challenging

(B) Clarification

(C) Paraphrasing

(D) Focusing


(127) General contraindications to medications include all but _____.

(A) Pregnancy

(B) Renal disease

(C) Allergies to the medicine

(D) Reduced body weight

(128) Regarding drug prescription to patients, which of the following is outside your purview as a nurse?

(A) Helping to prescribe drugs to patients

(B) Understanding the pharmacology of drugs and the pathology of the patient

(C) Discussing concerns about a prescription with the ordering physician

(D) Determining if the prescription is necessary based on the patient's pathology and the drug pharmacology

(129) Which of the following would classify as an immediate life-threatening adverse reaction?

(A) Difficult breathing following drug administration

(B) Visual impairment following drug administration

(C) Lip swelling following drug administration

(D) Phocomelia seen in infants resulting in short limbs after administration of thalidomide in pregnancy

(130) Concerning blood types, which is incorrect?

(A) Blood type O is a universal recipient.

(B) Blood type AB is a universal recipient.

(C) Blood type O is a universal donor.

(D) AA is a common genotype.

(131) All of the following are blood products except _____.

(A) Cryoprecipitate

(B) Packed blood cells

(C) Erythrocyte sediment

(D) Platelets

(132) A patient with severe anemia is being transfused and 30 minutes later, he is noticed to be febrile and tachycardic. What will be your next line of action?

(A) Stop the transfusion and inform the doctor.

(B) Continue the transfusion, give corticosteroids and antihistamines and inform the doctor.

(C) Stop the transfusion, give normal saline and inform the doctor.

(D) Continue the transfusion, give normal saline, antihistamines and corticosteroids and inform the doctor.

(133) A patient with blood type O receives type B blood. What type of reaction will occur?

(A) Allergic blood reaction

(B) Delayed hypersensitivity reaction

(C) Hemolytic transfusion reaction

(D) The blood types are compatible

(134) Which of these is true of central venous lines?

(A) They should be flushed daily with heparin.

(B) They should be flushed daily with warfarin.

(C) They should be flushed daily with normal saline.

(D) They should be flushed daily with protamine.

(135) Which of these should not be given via venous lines?

(A) Parenteral nutrition

(B) Chemotherapy

(C) Enteral nutrition

(D) Blood

(136) A patient had peripheral venous access one day ago, and during the administration of vancomycin, the patient complained of intense pain and heat in the arm. Pain subsided afterward, and upon administration of sterile injection water, there was no pain. What is the nurse's next line of action?

(A) Remove IV access to prevent infection.

(B) Reassure the patient and inform the doctor.

(C) Do nothing.

(D) None of the above.


(137) Which of the following is very important?

(A) Understanding the conversion of different metric systems in mathematics

(B) Understanding the relevant clinical metrics in drug administration

(C) Estimating figures of dosages

(D) Understanding brand dosage

(138) What is the conversion factor between grams (gr) and milligrams (mg)?

(A) 1 gr = 100 mg

(B) 1 gr = 10 mg

(C) 1 gr = 1 mg

(D) 1 gr = 1000 mg

(139) All of the following are unique procedures some patients may need to be trained on, except _____.

(A) Using an inhaler

(B) Taking insulin

(C) Administering tube feedings

(D) Checking the medication label

(140) What information should be checked on a medication label before administration?

(A) Name of the medication

(B) Dose of the medication

(C) Expiry date of the medication

(D) All of the above

(141) A 23-year-old student has just been discharged home from the ward following an episode of severe acute asthma. Which training will the patient benefit from?

(A) Inhaler technique

(B) Taking insulin

(C) Self-administering tube feeding

(D) Giving intramuscular injections

(142) What are some complications associated with total parenteral nutrition?

(A) Improved athletic performance ✗

(B) Faster recovery from surgery ✗

(C) Convenience

(D) Infection, sepsis, liver dysfunction and metabolic imbalances ✗

(143) How do nurses help manage pain in patients?

(A) By ignoring the pain

(B) By distracting patients from the pain ⟶ 2

(C) By administering pain medication ✓

(D) By telling patients to endure the pain ✗

(144) What are non-opioids used for in pain management?

(A) Mild pain ✓

(B) Moderate to severe pain

(C) Chronic pain

(D) Emotional pain

(145) What is the role of nonpharmacological pain management techniques?

(A) To provide immediate pain relief

(B) To eliminate the need for pain medication

(C) To distract patients from pain

(D) To improve patient satisfaction

(146) What is the importance of proper pain management?

(A) To prevent patients from seeking medical attention

(B) To avoid the need for pain medication

(C) To promote patient comfort and well-being

(D) To encourage patients to endure pain without intervention

(147) How should opioid medications be tapered or discontinued?

(A) Abruptly

(B) When the patient requests it

(C) Based on the health care provider's discretion.

(D) In a gradual and supervised manner

(148) What is the best location for the nurse to use for intravenous therapy?

(A) Most distant veins on the nondominant hand

(B) Hand veins

(C) Upper limbs

(D) Lower limbs


(149) What are some potential consequences of fluid overload in intravenous therapy?

(A) Hematoma and phlebitis

(B) Allergic reactions and anaphylaxis

(C) Infections and emboli

(D) Edema and respiratory distress

(150) A two-year-old boy was brought into the children's emergency department with a history of seven episodes of vomiting and nine episodes of the passage of loose stool over the past 24 hours, with signs of severe dehydration. What is the most appropriate route for resuscitation in this patient?

(A) Oral route

(B) Intramuscular route

(C) Intravenous route

(D) Transdermal route

## Test 1: Answers and Explanations

(1) (D) Legal documentation on how clients should be handled if they are unable to communicate.

Advance directives refer to legal documentation that clearly states the wishes of patients about their care if they become unable or incapacitated to communicate. Some advance directives include living wills, health care proxies/durable power of attorneys for health care and the Uniform Anatomical Gift Act.

(2) (D) All of the above.

If an individual has prepared advance directives, the nurse should document this in the patient's records. Other relevant health care personnel should be informed and the directives should be strictly adhered to as occasions arise. If these documents have not been prepared, the nurse can counsel the patient on the need to prepare them.

(3) (B) Tasks that require lower levels of professional judgment.

The nature of the task will determine if it can be delegated or not. Some tasks involve client needs that follow set routines and require lower levels of professional judgment and competence. Such tasks can be easily delegated. But there are other tasks that involve meeting the needs of clients who are in dynamic or unstable conditions. Here, there can be rapid changes requiring quick judgment calls and higher competence. Such tasks should not be delegated.

(4) (B) Person, task, circumstance, direction, supervision.

The right person asks: *Is this the person right for the task?*
 The right task asks: *Is this a task to be delegated?*
The right circumstance asks: *What is the state of the patient?* The right direction/communication asks: *Is there a clear and detailed explanation of the task to be performed?*
The right supervision asks: *Who will be held accountable for the outcome of this task?*

(5) (D) Retrospective reimbursement.

In the retrospective reimbursement system, health care facilities receive payments for the care they render based on the cost, and insurance companies pay for all the services irrespective of the cost.

(6) (A) Individualization.

The plan that is developed for each patient must be individualized based on the patient's condition and need. This means that a nurse cannot make general health care plans for patients, even when they have similar diagnoses. No two bodies are the same, and individuals will always be unique in their physiology, their reactions, actions and adaptations.

(7) (A) Apologize to the client and allow him to view his records.

Patients have a right to speak privately to their health care providers and have their information treated confidentially. They have the right to look through their medical records and request an amendment of any inaccurate information. You should apologize to the client and allow him to view his records. Later, in private, you can speak to the staff about the rights of the patient.

(8) (D) All of the above.

All clients have a right to choose the health care provider they want. They also have the right to choose the type of health care plans that they want and those that they do not want. This bill allows them to accept or reject interventions, no matter how essential health care personnel know they are.

(9) (D) Playing multiple roles for effectiveness.

Advocacy to other staff means updating other nursing staff members about client advocacy and how this role should be seamlessly integrated into their practice. It should also include documenting or orally communicating the client's needs to other staff members. It includes utilizing advocacy resources efficiently. Playing multiple roles is not part of efficacy, as all health care personnel have specialized training.

(10) (D) B and C.

The nurse must assess the patient before arriving at the diagnosis and recognizing the client's need. Once a need for referral is recognized, the RN should contact the appropriate external resource that can meet the needs of the client. The external resources in the scenario presented are the psychologist, the psychotherapist and the physician.

(11) (D) Circulation, airway, breathing.

The ABCs of resuscitation mean airway, breathing and cardiovascular or circulatory system. This is useful in deciding where to start attending to a patient who has undergone a cardiac arrest. However, it is crucial to note that the recent update has changed the sequence to CAB, meaning chest compressions come first, followed by airway and then breathing.

(12) (C) One where mistakes are seen as opportunities for improvement.

A blameless or blame-free environment is required for performance improvement. A blameless environment is one where mistakes are seen as opportunities for improvement. In this type of environment, the focus is not on the individual who made a mistake but on the different ways to improve the processes and workflow and make it fail-safe.

(13) (A) Core measures.

Core measures refer to standard measurements of quality. They are developed by the JCAHO (Joint Commission on the Accreditation of Health Care Organizations). They evaluate values like the population of clients on the ward, specific diseases (such as pneumonia or sepsis) and organizational measures.

(14) (D) None of the above.

All methods of performance improvement have the following in common: problem definition, relevant data collection, analysis of collected data, root cause analysis, generating possible solutions or alternatives, narrowing down to a solution or alternative with the greatest feasibility and highest chance of success and evaluation of the effectiveness of the implemented solution.

(15) (B) RNs.

RNs are licensed health care personnel who are trained to deliver nursing care in health care settings. They can manage both stable and unstable patients in structured or unstructured environments. They are also trained to coordinate other nursing team members, such as nursing assistants and LPNs.

(16) (D) Social workers.

Social workers ensure that the client is appropriately moved in the continuum of care and that there is no deficit after the patient is discharged. They are also essential in cases of child abuse, neglect or malpractice and can provide a much-needed link and support for victims.

(17) (C) Conceptualization.

At this point, those affected by the conflict begin to understand what is happening and why it happened. They begin to provide logical or illogical reasons that they believe have brought them to that position.

(18) (C) Avoidance, accommodating without addressing issues, competition.

Avoidance: Prolonged withdrawal and avoidance of the entire situation are unhealthy.
Competition: Competition is very unhealthy for the health care team when it stems from conflict.
Accommodating others without addressing issues: While it is good to be accommodating and considerate, issues that are important to the individual should be resolved.

(19) (D) Teenager, young man, middle-aged man, elderly woman.

The teenager is experiencing an acute symptom that can be resolved within seconds by stopping the transfusion and administering an antipyretic. Then the nurse should attend to the patient from the auto crash to prevent him from going into shock. Then the nurse should attend to the middle-aged man who is in pain. The chemo patient is most likely stable at this point.

(20) (C) Race.

Race has nothing to do with establishing priorities in patient care. Any racial discrimination is a crime and can make health care personnel liable for litigation. Racial discrimination is a very serious offense, and it is not tolerated in health care practitioners. Priorities should be based on an understanding of the pathophysiology of the disease condition and presentation to know who needs more urgent care.

(21) (C) Recovery of client.

The ultimate determinant of the effectiveness of care is the recovery of the client.

(22) (B) Ethical standards conflict with client interests.

Many times, ethical dilemmas come into play when an action might be in the client's interest but is not in line with the ethical standards of practice. Nurses must not have any clash of beliefs with ethical standards. Whatever opinions they have should have been long addressed before the point of care delivery to the client.

(23) (A) It helps nurses to better commit to their responsibilities.

For nurses to understand the need to commit to their responsibility in the health space and society at large, it is nonnegotiable that evaluation of planned outcomes should take place. The role that a nurse has played in providing quality care without prejudice must be assessed and reported for further research or review.

(24) (D) 09/10/20 1145 hrs. IM diclofenac 75 mg STAT given. Patient reports pain as 2/10.

The right way to input information for clients is the date, time, drug and correct route of administration, dose frequency and assessment of the patient.

(25) (C) "I am sorry, Joe. I can't give you that information."

Let Joe know that you cannot give out such information. HIPAA protects the client's personal information, such as name, date of birth, social security number, diagnosis and treatment. This act ensures that those who have access to the information are involved in the management or care of the patient.

(26) (D) B and C.

Blind patients can hear, so they can be communicated with orally. Braille is a system of reading and writing that utilizes tactile representation of letters of the alphabet using raised dots. It is used by blind people or those with poor vision. In the health care setting, it can be used effectively to communicate with blind clients by those trained in its use.

(27) (D) "I cannot give the medication because you did not document it. Verbal orders are recognized only during emergencies. I suggest you ask another physician to come document it."

Verbal orders should not be used except in case of emergency, and a nurse is one of those responsible for maintaining order in the health care setting. If an order is given and not documented and anything goes wrong, the nurse will be liable because it was not documented. So the question should be, "Who gave the order?"

(28) (D) B and C.

Target screening can be done when some people show strong tendencies, signs or symptoms of a particular condition or disease. This target screening is also done when a client is at risk of a certain ailment or needs to rule out a possible condition.

(29) (D) Help clients express themselves more.

The purpose of a health history is to gather information about the patient's health status. This involves the use of open-ended questions (Option A) to gather broad subjective information, and closed-ended questions (Option B) to gather specific factual details. Interview-style questions (Option C) are often used in health history to engage in dialogue with the client. Therefore, these all are parts of a health history. However, a health history does not inherently help clients express themselves more (Option D), as it is focused on collecting information related to their health, not on improving their communication or self-expression skills.

(30) (D) All of the above.

A patient who has been having regular unprotected sex can be counseled on abstinence, sticking to a partner or using condoms to reduce the risk of contracting STIs. Nurses can also counsel patients on the need to use contraception to prevent unwanted or unplanned pregnancies.

(31) (A) Educating the parents about a balanced diet.

In a family with children, the parents are usually responsible for feeding the children. Therefore, counseling them is very important for the children to have a balanced diet.

(32) (A) Internal locus.

Locus of control refers to the point where an individual's control or power over the future lies. In some people, the locus of control is internal. In others, it is external. When it is internal, individuals believe they have control over their own future and whatever troubles they might encounter. When it is external, individuals believe that the future and all it brings is beyond their abilities to impact.

(33) (D) All of the above.

Assessments can also be structured and formal questions. They can be set surveys or interviews. Assessments can also be made by observing the behavior of patients.

(34) (B) Infants.

This stage also coincides with Piaget's first phase of cognitive development in children, known as the sensorimotor stage. Children learn about their surroundings through their sensory and motor activities at this stage.

(35) (D) All of the above.

While the question does not provide specific details about the child's behavior, it mentions that the child has started to challenge the mother's authority at home. Given this information, it is important to counsel the mother on helping her child avoid potential risks. The options provided include smoking, unsupervised swimming and falls. These are common risks that children may face, and it is essential to educate parents on how to prevent these hazards and ensure the child's safety.

(36) (A) Care of children and aging parents.

Individuals in this stage are middle-aged adults. Adults at this stage are concerned with a need to produce structures, people and things that will outlive them. They have various worries, ranging from childcare to aging parents' care. They are also concerned about diagnoses of chronic health conditions and worry about their impact on the world.

(37) (B) Prescription medications.

Hepatic changes will result in reduced hepatic blood flow and metabolism, leading to reduced hepatic clearance and a subsequent increase in the concentrations of medications in the body.

(38) (D) None of the above.

The most accurate method of determining the EDD is through an ultrasound scan done in the first trimester of pregnancy. The LMP is limited because the mother might not recall the exact date, and the cycle might not be exact. Ultrasound done after the first trimester is not as accurate. The ovulation date is also not reliable.

(39) (C) Delivery of the fetus.

The second stage of labor is from full cervical dilatation (10 cm) to delivery of the fetus. Braxton-Hicks contractions occur during the first stage of labor, usually during the latent phase. Here mild or minor contractions happen, but cervical dilatation is less than 4 cm.

(40) (C) Warm water.

Alcohol should not be used to clean the umbilical cord as it has been found that it can irritate the skin, delay healing and delay the stump from falling off. Warm water is now recommended several times a day. Other parts of the baby should also be cleaned.

(41) (A) Difficulty breathing.

Common allergic reaction symptoms include but are not limited to swelling, numbness, itching or tingling at the exposure point, breathing difficulties, rashes or bumps, hypotension and tachycardia. Swelling, numbness or tingling sensations around the lips, mouth or tongue usually indicate extremely serious allergic reactions.

(42) (B) Document the client's allergic reaction for future purposes.

Every allergic reaction must be documented to inform future health care measures. The substance that the patient reacted to, the dose of the substance and what was done to arrest the situation should be clearly documented. The patient should also be duly informed about what caused the reaction.

(43) (B) A 30-year-old sedated and unrestrained patient.

The 30-year-old sedated and unrestrained client is more prone to falls and injuries than other clients. While factors like age and mental state can make clients more prone to falls and injuries, other factors such as level of consciousness, muscular strength and impaired reaction time are also high-risk factors.

(44) (D) They are 4'9" or 80 pounds.

Car seat laws and requirements for infants and children can vary by state. However, most laws require that infants and toddlers be strapped in car seats until they are 4'9" or 80 pounds.

(45) (B) Having oxygen and suction equipment on standby at all times.

Preventive measures for patients at risk of seizures include identifying and removing environmental triggers, lowering the client's bed or having the mattress placed on the floor and having oxygen and suction equipment at the client's bedside at all times.

(46) (C) Using one distinct identifier alongside the room number of clients for easy and efficient identification.

It is recommended to have at least two distinct identifiers aside from the room number of clients. Room numbers in themselves should not be used as unique identifiers. Rather, nurses should consider using patients' full names, complete dates of birth and other unique identification codes.

(47) (B) Yes.

RNs should verify the appropriateness and accuracy of each treatment order, especially when any appear out of place or questionable. Nurses should contact the health care personnel who have prescribed such treatment or procedure for proper verification.

(48) (A) Code Gray is the appropriate code for communicating infant abduction.

This is false. Code Blue is a code name for cardiac arrest. Other common codes included Code Red for fire, Code Orange for a chemical spill, Code Pink for an infant abduction and Code Gray for a hurricane, cyclone or severe weather storm.

(49) (C) None of the above.

Use your arms and legs muscles to lift, not your back. Also, provide a secure base for supporting yourself while lifting by keeping your feet apart. The muscles of the back should not be used to lift.

red → fire

pink → child obduction

orange → Chemical

grey → Natural disaster

blue → art heart

(50) (D) The developmental stage of the client and the environment.

Every assistive device assigned to a patient must be properly suited to meet individual needs, such as cognitive ability, muscular strength, developmental stage, height, weight and environment. Other factors, such as the distance of the client's home, cultural and religious affiliations and income level, do not play a significant role in determining the client's ability to use an assistive device.

(51) (D) Dispose of biohazardous material in any trash can available.

Disposal of biohazardous material in any trash can is inappropriate and dangerous. A general principle for handling biohazardous waste is to properly dispose of it following stipulated national, state and local laws.

(52) (D) All of the above.

Some situations nurses should look out for when inspecting equipment include frayed electrical cords, overloaded power outlets, loose or missing equipment parts and other questionable conditions that could threaten the client care environment.

(53) (C) Participate in periodic training and mock drills.

A key way for RNs to prepare for security threats is to go for periodic training and review policies and procedures for ensuring security before any breach occurs.

(54) (A) Airborne, contact, droplet and vector borne.

The mode of transmission is the specific medium through which the infectious agent is transmitted from the reservoir to a new host. Modes of transmission of pathogens are contact (direct and indirect), airborne, droplet and vector-borne. When pathogens leave through the portal of exit of a reservoir, they are borne through these mediums until they gain access to the portal of entry of a new host.

(55) (C) Getting bitten by a mosquito carrying the West Nile virus.

Vector-borne transmission occurs when an insect or other animal spreads a pathogen. In this case, the mosquito acts as a vector, carrying the West Nile virus from one host to another.

(56) (D) All of the above.

Handwashing should be done before and after contact with a client, before and after removing gloves, after touching equipment, instruments and other treatment materials with bare hands, and when hands have been soiled with bodily fluids, secretions and chemicals.

(57) (A) Measures taken to prevent the transfer of disease-causing organisms from one person or object to the other.

Aseptic techniques are measures taken in addition to standard and transmission-based precautions to prevent the transfer of disease-causing organisms from one person or object to the other. Aseptic techniques include barriers, patient and equipment preparation, environmental controls and contact guidelines.

(58) (B) Reports should go to the Centers for Disease Control and Prevention.

Reports about communicable diseases, epidemics and other outbreaks should be submitted to the Centers for Disease Control and Prevention.

(59) (B) Ensure that staff members adhere to infection control measures.

RNs should watch out for themselves and other staff members to ensure they adhere to good infection control and prevention measures.

(60) (A) The patient's level of consciousness.

Every restraint or safety device used must be appropriate for every situation and should not increase the risk of accidents or harmful situations. It's important to consider the patient's level of consciousness to ensure that the restraint or safety device doesn't cause further harm.

(61) (D) BMI.

A patient's vital signs include blood pressure, pulse rate, respiratory rate and body temperature. These four signs signify the body's most basic function. The Body Mass Index (BMI) is a measure of the body's weight-to-height ratio. It is used to divide people into normal, overweight and obese. It is calculated as weight/height $^2$.

(62) (A) Korotkoff sounds.

Korotkoff sounds are produced by the blood pressure cuff and heard with a stethoscope when checking for blood pressure. They are produced as the cuff compresses the brachial artery and causes turbulent blood flow in the artery. The sounds are divided into five phases.

(63) (D) A and B.

Before performing any test, it is necessary to confirm the doctor's order for the tests and that the right patient is getting the test. This can be done by checking the order that was documented by the doctor. The next step is to ask the patient to say their name and then crosscheck that it is the same patient that the order was written for.

(64) (A) Electrical impulses of the heart.

The ECG records the electrical activities of the heart. It shows the velocity of the heartbeat, its consistency or rhythmicity and how strong the electrical impulses are as they move from chamber to chamber in the heart.

(65) (D) None of the above.

All the methods listed can be used to obtain blood samples. Arterial sampling collects blood from arteries, venipuncture obtains blood from superficial veins and dermal puncture obtains blood from the fingertips.

(66) (D) Needle prick.

Venipuncture is a routine procedure carried out in the hospital. However, it has its complications. The patient is at risk of infection from a contaminated cannula. There's also the risk of injury to the skin, excessive bleeding and delayed wound healing. The nurse is at risk of needle pricks. Needle pricks predispose nurses to infections like hepatitis and retroviral disease.

(67) (B) Apply pressure on the sample collection site.

To prevent hematoma formation at the sample collection site during a venipuncture, pressure should be applied with gauze for a few minutes until blood flow stops. A hematoma happens when blood leaks from the vein into the surrounding tissues. It is most identifiable by swelling.

(68) (D) Conscious patients.

Patients with nasogastric feeding tubes are at risk of aspiration of oropharyngeal or gastrointestinal secretions. Patients with an impaired gag or cough reflex find it challenging to expel contaminants in the airway, so the contaminants stray into the lungs and block the airway. Sedated patients are also at risk of aspiration.

(69) (A) Hypovolemic shock.

Hypovolemic shock occurs when there is a depletion of blood fluids, which leads to a reduction in tissue perfusion. The endothelial cells experience ischemia because they are deprived of oxygen, and endothelial cell apoptosis occurs. The most common cause of hypovolemic shock is hemorrhage.

(70) (D) All of the above.

Patients who are malnourished and don't eat a balanced diet have a chance of skin breakdown because the nutrients to strengthen the connective skin tissues are absent. They also have a weak immune system and are prone to infections.

(71) (D) CT scan.

Infections can present with a persistent fever that might resist antipyretics and tepid sponging. A blood culture might be required to detect the presence of microorganisms. A complete blood count would also be useful. A CT scan would not be routinely ordered for a patient with persistent fever.

(72) (D) All of the above.

The quantity of drainage is measured and documented. The nature and color, if it is bilious or coffee-ground colored, might indicate that there is internal bleeding.

(73) (C) A few inches above the selected site.

The tourniquet is placed about four to five inches above the selected site. The purpose of the tourniquet is to block blood flow for a short period so that the vein is engorged and more visible for the insertion of the cannula.

(74) (C) A and B.

The catheter is inserted into the urethral meatus and advanced through the urethra above the point when urine is seen in the urine catheter. However, the catheter can also be inserted through the skin, at the pubic region into the bladder, by suprapubic cystostomy. This usually happens when the urethra is not patent.

(75) (B) Olfactory nerve.

The olfactory nerve is the first cranial nerve, and it is involved in smell. The nasal cavity contains more than 100 million olfactory receptors. These receptors are stimulated by molecules from different substances, then stimulate other fibers, which eventually stimulate the olfactory nerve.

(76) (C) Polydipsia.

Hypoglycemia commonly presents with lethargy, sweating, clumsiness, loss of consciousness, coma and even death. Hyperglycemia presents with polydipsia (increased thirst) because there is an increased level of glucose in the blood. This increase leads to a high osmotic concentration of the blood, leading to dehydration, and this sends a signal to the brain to stimulate thirst.

(77) (A) Regional, general.

Anesthesia can be regional/local or general/systemic. Regional anesthesia is usually preferable because of the side effects and risks of general anesthesia.

(78) (B) Epidural.

Epidural anesthesia is a form of regional anesthesia where an anesthetic is injected into the epidural space above the dura mater. It is used during abdominal or lower limb surgeries or procedures. It is also given to women in labor who do not want to experience labor pains.

(79) (A) External.

External insults can be foreign bodies or microorganisms introduced into the body system from the exterior. External insults can result in internal injury. So the gunshot is an external injury that eventually results in internal injury.

(80) (B) Breakdown of RBCs.

Bilirubin is formed from the breakdown of red blood cells. RBCs are broken down into heme and globin. Globin is broken into amino acids, while heme is further broken down into iron and biliverdin. The iron is reused and recycled while the biliverdin is converted to the unconjugated form of bilirubin, which is transported to the liver bound to albumin.

(81) (D) All of the above.

Just like any procedure, the patient must give informed consent. The procedure must be thoroughly explained to the patient. The environment must be sterile and aseptic techniques must be employed.

(82) (B) To reduce the breathing workload on the patient.

Ventilators reduce the breathing workload on the patient. The patient is intubated with an endotracheal tube that is appropriate for the age and procedure. The tube delivers the oxygen, which is also connected to the mechanical ventilator.

(83) (C) Artificial aspiration of pulmonary secretions.

Suctioning is the mechanical aspiration of pulmonary secretions from the airways. It is usually done in unconscious or sedated patients. Its purpose is to prevent secretions from blocking the airways or being aspirated into the trachea and lungs, which can lead to death.

(84) (D) None of the above.

Povidone is a good antiseptic, notable for drying wounds fast. Methylated spirit is useful for dressing, and honey has been noted to prevent bacterial infection and promote rapid healing, especially for open wounds. These all help to lower the rate of surgical site infection.

(85) (A) Examine vital signs.

A patient recovering from general anesthesia is at risk of dysphagia and laryngospasms. The patient is monitored after surgery by the nurse. The vital signs are first examined. The pulse rate and blood pressure are measured. The respiratory system is also examined.

(86) (D) Coughing and postural drainage.

Simple techniques for pulmonary hygiene include coughing, deep breathing and postural drainage. Advanced techniques include percussion and vibrations.

(87) (B) Openings from the outside to the inside.

Ostomies are surgical operations that create openings from the outside to the inside. They can be done to divert the bowels, such as through a colostomy.

(88) (A) Peritonitis.

Peritonitis is the inflammation of the abdominal cavity. Technically, it is the serosal membrane of the abdominal cavity and the organ it contains that is inflamed. It usually presents with fever, abdominal pain, diarrhea, ascites, and there might be ileus and diarrhea. There is also usually a history of recent abdominal surgery or previous history of peritonitis and immunosuppressive agents or diseases.

(89) (A) Upper limb.

The AV graft is a connection between an artery and a vein that is used in dialysis. The upper limb is the routine position for the graft, even though the lower limb can also be used when necessary.

(90) (D) Mercury.

Mercury is toxic to the human body. It is not an electrolyte. Sodium is the most dominant extracellular ion, and it helps in muscle contraction. Calcium helps with bone strengthening and cardiac contractions. Magnesium also plays a role in preventing the continuous contraction of muscles.

(91) (D) EUCR, hyperkalemia.

Hyperkalemia is an elevation of the potassium levels in the blood above the expected standard value. Features of hyperkalemia include muscle paralysis, generalized body weakness, nausea and cardiac arrhythmias. Therefore, this patient should be screened for hyperkalemia.

(92) (A) Diuretics.

Hyponatremia is the reduction in the sodium level in the body below the usual standard. Thyroid gland diseases, renal failure and diuretic medications can cause hyponatremia. Both loop and thiazide diuretics are known to cause hyponatremia by inhibiting the absorption of sodium and stimulating sodium excretion respectively.

(93) (C) Shock.

Hypovolemia is a reduction in the fluid in the blood. Hypovolemic shock occurs when there is a depletion of blood fluids, which leads to a reduction in tissue perfusion. This deficit in fluid in the blood volume and reduction of tissue perfusion can lead to shock, reduced cardiac output, coma and death.

(94) (C) Ringer's lactate.

Blood volume expanders are intravenous fluids that can help to increase or maintain blood volume. They are usually important in conditions like hypovolemic shock or in surgery when there is anticipation of blood or fluid loss. Normal saline can also be used.

(95) (B) Continuous monitoring and recording of an ECG.

Telemetry is continuously monitoring and recording the ECG strips. It is mostly done by a telemetry technician, but nurses can monitor telemetry too.

(96) (D) A and C.

Hemothorax refers to the presence of blood in the pleural space. The patient might be breathless, and there might be reduced breath sounds, chest rise and percussion notes on the affected site. Depending on the extent of the bleeding, there might be marked hemodynamic changes.

(97) (C) A and B.

Arterial lines can be placed in the femoral, brachial and radial arteries. These lines are inserted via a surgical procedure to monitor the patient's blood pressure. Arterial lines can also be used to obtain frequent blood samples.

(98) (A) Spirometry.

Patients with impaired ventilation/oxygenation should be assessed with pulmonary function tests like pulse oximetry, spirometry, lung compliance and forced vital capacity.

(99) (D) B and C.

It is expedient that patients know what to look out for when they are at home. They should be able to recognize symptoms of a condition, what to do and when to report to the hospital promptly.

(100) (D) Visual assessment.

Patients with a long history of diabetes are more prone to visual abnormalities such as cataracts, macular degeneration and glaucoma, among other ocular conditions. This patient being elderly potentiates the risk of visual abnormalities. Hence, the most appropriate assessment is a visual assessment. However, other basic care assessments should be carried out for all admitted patients.

(101) (B) Fecal impaction.

Fecal impaction is the collection of compressed or hardened feces in the colon or rectum, commonly occurring in older people. Prompt recognition and differentiation from other causes of the inability to pass stool are important in patient management.

(102) (C) Mobility issues can affect other systems aside from the musculoskeletal system.

Mobility issues can affect the respiratory, gastrointestinal and urinary systems. Mobility issues can be from genetic or acquired factors. Muscle contraction is usually graded on a scale of 0 to 5. Mobility issues are usually multifactorial, involving nerves, muscles, electrolytes and psychology.

(103) (D) Nonpharmacological comfort interventions can be effective in the management of pain.

Nonpharmacological comfort interventions, such as patient education, companionship and music, can effectively manage pain. Acute pain is usually described based on duration and not severity. Pharmacological treatment is not always effective in pain management, and severe cases may need interventional management rather than pharmacological. Pain can be a complication of treatment in oncology cases. However, symptoms and resolution of pain can usually be a sign of improvement following treatment.

(104) (C) Document for possible revision of medications and reduction of dosage.

Documentation for possible medication revision and dosage reduction is the next best course of action, as overdosing can cause excessive somnolence. Other answer options are inaccurate.

(105) (B) Use of a waterbed.

The use of a waterbed is most appropriate in this patient to prevent pressure sores due to the severe injuries limiting mobility. Other options will not prove as effective or may further worsen the patient's condition.

(106) (D) Suprapubic (bladder) massage.

Suprapubic (bladder) massage will not increase the rate of renal elimination of the toxic substance.

(107) (A) Increasing intravenous fluid intake.

Increasing intravenous fluid intake is not an appropriate part of the evaluation and care of this patient as it offers little care of the primary pathology unless other complications, such as dehydration, occur.

(108) (D) Encouraging ambulation.

Encouraging ambulation is an inappropriate line of care for this patient. Other options, such as the administration of antipyretics, tepid sponging, adequate exposure and increasing fluid intake, all aim to reduce the body temperature.

(109) (A) Sedate the patient.

Sedating the patient is an inappropriate line of care as it will affect the assessment of consciousness and mask neurological signs needed for patient evaluation. All other lines of care are appropriate for this patient.

(110) (D) Regular fasting.

Regular fasting is not advisable for this patient, who has previously been diagnosed with an eating disorder. All other counsel will benefit the patient and is adjuvant care in managing cholecystitis.

(111) (B) Spoon feed the patient while propped up in bed.

Spoon feeding of the patient while the patient is propped up in bed poses a high risk of aspiration.

(112) (B) History of maternal illness in pregnancy.

The history of maternal illness in pregnancy is the most inappropriate question in the evaluation of this patient as the child is past the neonatal period, and poor weight gain is likely related to the current diet and acquired factors.

(113) (A) Zimmer's walking frame.

Zimmer's walking frame is the best mobility assistive device for this patient as the weight is evenly distributed and reduces weight bearing on the post-op limb.

(114) (D) It cannot happen without dependence.

Substance abuse is defined as the overuse of a substance that is addictive or use that is not prescribed by qualified medical personnel. Substance abuse can lead to physical dependence, which happens when a person begins to experience adverse physical reactions to drug withdrawal. However, it is important to state that addiction can occur without physical dependence.

(115) (B) Addiction.

Addiction is the constant need for a person to take a particular substance despite obvious physical, mental and social or economic harm and a loss of control over the use of that substance. So even though Matt knows his smoking is affecting him, he still feels a need to keep smoking.

(116) (B) Evaluate the patient using CAGE-AID.

CAGE-AID is a standard test for evaluating clients with substance abuse disorder. Patients in this category might display hyperactivity or slow movements, tremors, poor hygiene, the presence of needle marks on upper and lower extremities and poor health status.

(117) (A) Interval follow-up evaluation, range of impaired functioning.

Two standard assessment tools are interval follow-up evaluation and range of impaired functioning.

(118) (C) Adventitious.

An adventitious crisis occurs during a major social disturbance. It includes natural disasters, war or terrorism. Developmental/maturational crises are predicted occurrences that happen in life. They occur due to growth. Situational crises refer to events that are unpredictable. They are random life events that happen to people.

(119) (C) Cultural care negation and accommodation

Leininger's transcultural nursing theory includes three major nursing decisions and actions:

Cultural preservation and maintenance (Option B) - helping the client to retain and/or preserve relevant care values so they can maintain their well-being, recover from illness, or face handicaps or death.

Cultural care accommodation/negotiation (Option C is incorrect because the term is 'negotiation', not 'negation') - helping the client adapt to or negotiate with others for a beneficial or satisfying health outcome.

Cultural care repatterning/restructuring (Option D) - assisting the client to reorder, change, or greatly modify their lifeways for new, different, and beneficial health care patterns.

Option A (Cultural interference and restructuring) is not a component of Leininger's transcultural nursing theory, making it the correct answer.

(120) (D) All of the above.

Needs might be adequate nutrition and fluids due to anorexia and dehydration. Patients might also have psychological needs which can be diverse. Some of these can be corrected, while others might have to be managed with the help of psychologists and family members.

(121) (D) A and B.

Ill health and disability are biological needs. Unemployment is a socioeconomic need.

(122) (A) Denial.

The Kübler-Ross model describes grief in five stages: denial, anger, bargaining, depression and acceptance. Denial is when the person refuses to accept the loss that has occurred.

(123) (A) Psychotic disorder.

Psychotic disorders include schizophrenia, schizotypal personality disorder and schizoaffective disorder.

(124) (D) B and C.

A nurse must attend to patients with a consciousness of their spiritual leanings and provide appropriate care for them without offending them.

(125) (A) Alarm.

The stage of alarm is where certain physiological responses show that there is an upset in the body's homeostasis. The resistance stage is marked by increased cardiac output and a maintained respiratory rate and blood pressure increase. Here, the body is trying to deal with the effect of the stress. The third stage is exhaustion; at this point, the body has used all its resources in trying to deal with the stress.

(126) (A) Challenging.

This means forcing clients to defend their choices and opinions. It is nontherapeutic and should be avoided. Clarification, paraphrasing and focusing are all therapeutic.

(127) (D) Reduced body weight.

Pregnancy, renal disease and allergy are all general contraindications to medications; however, reduced body weight is not a contraindication, as the dose can be recalculated for weight.

(128) (A) Helping to prescribe drugs to patients.

It is illegal for a nurse to prescribe medications for patients as only the doctor is licensed to do so, except in states where nurses have such licenses. It is important to understand the pharmacology and the patient's pathology as this will help determine if there is anything wrong with the prescription so it can be discussed with the doctor.

(129) (A) Difficult breathing following drug administration.

Difficult breathing is life-threatening as this can lead to tissue hypoxia and, consequently, death. Visual impairment is a very serious challenge but is not immediately life-threatening. Lip swelling is minor, and phocomelia, though an adverse reaction, is not immediately life-threatening.

(130) (A) Blood type O is a universal recipient.

Blood type A has A antigens, and blood type B has B antigens. AB has both A and B antigens, so it is a universal recipient as it cannot be transfused to any other blood type except AB. Blood type O has neither A nor B antigens, so an agglutination reaction will not occur since there is no antigen to react with. Hence blood type O is a universal donor.

(131) (C) Erythrocyte sediment.

Erythrocyte sediment is a measure of an active inflammatory process. Blood products are therapeutic substances derived from blood. The different blood products and their components are red blood cells, platelets, fresh frozen plasma, albumin, clotting factors, cryoprecipitate and whole blood.

(132) (C) Stop the transfusion, give normal saline and inform the doctor.

In case of a transfusion reaction, the best response is to stop the transfusion and give IV normal saline. Antihistamines and corticosteroids with antipyretics can also be given, and urine output should be monitored. A doctor should be informed. It is important to send a blood sample from the contralateral limb of the patient for regrouping and crossmatching.

(133) (C) Hemolytic transfusion reaction.

People with blood type O are universal donors and can give blood to any type, but they are only compatible to receive blood from other type O donors. If a person with type O blood receives type B blood, their body would identify the B antigens as foreign and would mount an immune response. This could result in a hemolytic transfusion reaction, where the immune system destroys the transfused blood cells. This is a serious and potentially life-threatening response. Therefore, ensuring blood compatibility is crucial in transfusions.

(134) (A) They should be flushed daily with heparin.

Central venous lines should be flushed daily and after every use with heparin to keep the line patent.

(135) (C) Enteral nutrition.

Enteral nutrition is taken by direct tubing to the intestine or can be ingested orally but is contraindicated for venous administration.

(136) (B) Reassure the patient and inform the doctor.

Reassure the patient and inform the doctor to determine the next line of action. It is a known fact that some medications are irritating to veins. Hence they should be administered slowly, and the patient should be reassured. However, if pain persists after administration, the IV line should be removed and another inserted.

(137) (B) Understanding the relevant clinical metrics in drug administration.

There are different metric concepts in mathematics, but some have more clinical significance. Estimation can be helpful but sometimes dangerous; for example, in the administration of chemotherapy, the slightest increase in dose can be lethal.

(138) (D) 1 gr = 1000 mg.

When converting from grams (gr) to milligrams (mg), the conversion factor is 1 gr = 1000 mg.

(139) (D) Checking the medication label.

Patients are taught to check medication labels, but it's not a unique procedure that requires special training.

(140) (D) All of the above.

The nurse is expected to verify the medication's name, dose, expiry date and technique for administering it before administration.

(141) (A) Inhaler technique.

The patient will benefit from learning the appropriate inhaler technique for maintenance therapy.

(142) (D) Infection, sepsis, liver dysfunction and metabolic imbalances.

Total parenteral nutrition (TPN) is a method of delivering nutrition directly into the bloodstream when oral or enteral nutrition is not possible or insufficient. While TPN can be beneficial in providing essential nutrients to patients, it is not without potential complications. Complications associated with TPN include the risk of infection, which can lead to sepsis, as well as liver dysfunction and metabolic imbalances.

(143) (C) By administering pain medication.

Nurses help manage pain primarily by administering pain medications to patients.

(144) (A) Mild pain.

Nonopioids are nonnarcotic analgesics that are used to manage mild pain. They are not typically used for moderate to severe or chronic pain, which may require stronger analgesics such as opioids. Nonopioids reduce pain and inflammation; examples of non-opioid drugs include NSAIDs.

(145) (B) To eliminate the need for pain medication.

Nonpharmacological pain management techniques can help eliminate the need for pain medications in some cases.

(146) (C) To promote patient comfort and well-being.

Proper pain management is important to promote patient comfort and well-being.

(147) (D) In a gradual and supervised manner.

Opioid medications are usually tapered or discontinued gradually and supervised to prevent withdrawal symptoms and other complications.

(148) (A) Most distant veins on the nondominant hand.

The most distant veins on the nondominant hand are the best for the nurse to use so that the patient can fully use the dominant hand.

(149) (D) Edema and respiratory distress.

Fluid overload can lead to edema (accumulation of excess fluids in the third space) and respiratory distress. Respiratory distress can result from the accumulation of fluids in the pleural space.

(150) (C) Intravenous route.

The intravenous route will be the most appropriate route for resuscitation of this patient as it can deliver fluids directly to the child's system without the risk of vomiting, which would likely occur in the oral route.

# Test 2 Questions

(1) Which advance directive allows the relatives of a deceased patient to decide to donate the patient's organs?

(A) Living will

(B) Uniform Anatomical Gift Act

(C) Health care proxy

(D) None of the above

(2) Which of the following is not a legal document?

(A) Value history

(B) Self-determination act

(C) Health care proxy

(D) Uniform Anatomical Gift Act

(3) A nurse in the ER must attend to two patients urgently. One of them is a 60-year-old female stroke patient who presented with left-sided weakness and is unconscious and awaiting the results of the CT scan. She also needs to be turned. The other is a 25-year-old diabetic type 1 patient who was rushed in unconscious, looking very dehydrated, and needs to be resuscitated. Which of the following tasks should be delegated?

(A) Turning the stroke patient

(B) Resuscitating the 25-year-old

(C) Both tasks can be delegated

(D) None of the above


(4) Which of the following is not involved in case management?

(A) Development of health care plans

(B) Implementation of health care plans

(C) Evaluation of health care plans

(D) None of the above

(5) What are the things that must be considered in developing a patient plan?

(A) Diagnosis

(B) Actual problems

(C) Potential problems

(D) All of the above

(6) What legislation protects the personal information of the client?

(A) Patient's Bill of Rights

(B) HIPAA

(C) Informed consent

(D) All of the above

(7) _____ is not a client's responsibility.

(A) Treating health care workers with respect

(B) Paying medical bills

(C) Providing inaccurate information about health status

(D) None of the above

(8) _____ is not part of advocacy.

(A) Sensitization

(B) Explaining diagnoses

(C) Education

(D) Rejecting or accepting intervention on behalf of the patient

(9) What is the first step in referring a client?

(A) Obtain necessary orders.

(B) Delegate.

(C) Assess the client.

(D) All of the above.

(10) In triaging, what skill is the RN required to have?

(A) Organization

(B) Time management

(C) Diagnosing

(D) All of the above

(11) Which skill must a nurse have to manage the workload effectively?

(A) Effective communication

(B) Systematic manner of work

(C) Knowledge of declining less urgent tasks

(D) All of the above

(12) A patient was transfused with two pints of whole blood and, after the second pint, had a severe transfusion reaction. What kind of event is this?

(A) Adverse drug reaction

(B) Sentinel event

(C) Auspicious event

(D) Tragic event

(13) What type of measures focus on the length of stay of 30 patients admitted for the same illness on the ward?

(A) Core measures

(B) Outcome measures

(C) Quality measures

(D) Quantity measures

(14) Which of the following traits must a nurse have to collaborate effectively with other health care professionals?

(A) High level of professionalism

(B) Sound judgment

(C) Good communication skills

(D) All of the above

(15) Why are interdisciplinary conferences important?

(A) For holistic management of patients

(B) For nurses to contribute to client care

(C) For nurses to learn from other health care disciplines

(D) All of the above

(16) At what stage of conflict does either party feel their needs are being sidelined or ignored?

(A) Action

(B) Conceptualization

(C) Anger

(D) Frustration

(17) What happens at the action stage of conflict?

(A) Both parties come to a resolution.

(B) Individuals respond to the frustrations and conclusions they have arrived at.

(C) A third party intervenes.

(D) All of the above.

(18) An unconscious 25-year-old man is rushed to the emergency room. A brief history from his relatives reveals that he is a known type I diabetic. He is still breathing. You perceive a fruity smell as you examine him. What is the most important investigation at this moment?

(A) Random blood glucose

(B) Urine

(C) CBC

(D) Fasting blood glucose

(19) How often should the plan of care be revised?

(A) Daily

(B) Weekly

(C) As often as needed

(D) Seldom

(20) Which of the following statements is true?

(A) Ethical dilemmas can be avoided in nursing care.

(B) Ethical dilemmas cannot be avoided in nursing care.

(C) Adhering to ethical standards will never go against the client's interests.

(D) None of the above.

(21) Why is the code of ethics important to the nursing profession?

(A) To provide a framework for decision making

(B) To provide responsibility reminders for nurses

(C) To control nurses' behavior

(D) A and B

(22) What must happen in the nursing profession as development occurs globally?

(A) The code of ethics must be abandoned.

(B) The code of ethics must be revised.

(C) The foundations of nursing must be revisited.

(D) The code of ethics should become a matter of personal conviction.


(23) What is the right way to input information for clients?

(A) 11/12/20 0830 hrs. Acetaminophen 900 mg STAT given. Pain has subsided.

(B) 11/12/20 0830 hrs. Acetaminophen 900 mg total dose given. Pain is reported as 2/10.

(C) 11/12/20 0830 hrs. Acetaminophen given. The patient is feeling better.

(D) 11/12/20 0830 hrs. IV Acetaminophen 900 mg STAT given. The patient reports pain as 5/10.

(24) A patient's relative asks to see the health records of her friend, who is also in the hospital. What should be your response?

(A) "I cannot allow that!"

(B) "I am sorry; I cannot allow you to see that."

(C) "Speak to your friend about it."

(D) All of the above


(25) A patient being discharged asked to take a look at her medical records. What should be your response?

(A) "Here they are; take a look."

(B) "Here is my password; check on the system."

(C) "I am not permitted to do that."

(D) "I will get you a copy from the records office."

(26) An order was documented for a medication to be given to the client QDS. What does this mean?

(A) As often as needed

(B) 4 times daily

(C) 3 times daily

(D) Twice daily

(27) A woman has just suffered a TIA. Which of the following acts would be termed as negligence?

(A) Admitting the patient

(B) Administering alteplase

(C) Not asking for a physiotherapist

(D) Not evaluating the patient for stroke

(28) Which of the following clients would require target screening?

(A) A 45-year-old man presenting for his routine check-up

(B) A 50-year-old man presenting with acute rhinitis

(C) A five-year-old boy whose weight for his age is below normal

(D) B and C

(29) One critical trait that a nurse must have while taking a detailed history is to be _____.

(A) Nonjudgmental

(B) Sentimental

(C) Attached

(D) Detached


(30) _____ is not a high-risk behavior.

(A) Excessive sun exposure

(B) Drug abuse

(C) Lack of sleep

(D) Exercise


(31) Readiness to learn is divided into _____ types

(A) 5

(B) 2

(C) 3

(D) 4

(32) Examples of barriers to learning do not include _____.

(A) Cultural and spiritual beliefs

(B) Literacy

(C) Language

(D) Rain

(33) A term neonate had an APGAR score of 6 in 1. What does this mean?

(A) Severely distressed, needs urgent intensive care

(B) Moderately distressed, needs moderate resuscitation

(C) In excellent condition

(D) In good condition

(34) What is expected in Erikson's second stage of development?

(A) Feeding every two hours

(B) Separation anxiety

(C) Hopping around

(D) Mastering toilet training

(35) Adolescents are in the identity vs. confusion stage. What should you not expect at this stage?

(A) Attraction toward the opposite sex

(B) Decreased self-consciousness

(C) Peer group acceptance

(D) None of the above

(36) Among the elderly, what are some things to expect?

(A) Living retrospectively

(B) Gradual decline in physical function

(C) Seeking purpose

(D) A and B

(37) _____ is not a part of the active management of the third stage of labor.

(A) 10 IU oxytocin

(B) Controlled cord traction

(C) Uterine massage

(D) Placenta separation

(38) What equipment is used to monitor the fetal heart rate?

(A) Sphygmomanometer

(B) Fetal heart Doppler

(C) Ultrasound scan

(D) All of the above


(39) One major way of detecting fetal distress in labor is through _____.

(A) Elevated fetal respiratory rate

(B) Decreased fetal movement

(C) Decreased uterine contractions

(D) Elevated fetal heart rate

(40) A 35-year-old patient, gravida 4, para 0, 4 alive, presents with significant blood loss following a spontaneous vaginal delivery (SVD). Based on your assessment of the number of soaked pads, the estimated blood loss exceeds 500 ml. What is the diagnosis?

(A) Disseminated intravascular coagulation

(B) Postpartum hemorrhage |

(C) Postpartum psychosis

(D) All of the above

(41) Assessing the client care environment involves taking into consideration factors such as _____.

(A) Luxury and distance ✓

(B) Age and income level

(C) Comfort and safety

(D) All of the above

(42) Which of the following is false about assessing the client care environment?

(A) Privacy is not a factor of concern when assessing the client care environment.

(B) Assessing the client care environment is a continuous process.

(C) The emotional, social and cultural preferences of the client should be considered.

(D) None of the above


(43) Which of the following helps in promoting staff safety?

(A) Providing education and training

(B) Creating a safe and ideal work environment

(C) Encouraging staff communication

(D) All of the above


(44) Clients who are unable to change their positions by themselves should be turned _____.

(A) Every 12 hours

(B) Every 2 hours

(C) Every 1 hour

(D) Every 6 hours

302

(45) Which of the following clients could be at a higher risk of identification errors?

(A) An unconscious patient

(B) A client in a public ward housing more than two patients

(C) A patient whose name and last name are the same

(D) A patient who cannot communicate in English


(46) Nurses must be prepared to handle emergencies _____.

(A) Only when they are internal disasters

(B) Especially when they are disease outbreaks

(C) Irrespective of where they occur and who is affected

(D) When their clients are at high risk of being impacted, whether at home or in the client care environment

(47) Which client category should be first recommended for discharge after treatment?

(A) Unstable clients

(B) Ambulatory clients

(C) Conscious clients

(D) It depends on the unique situation

(48) Why is communicating discreetly but effectively during disasters and other emergencies recommended?

(A) To prevent sabotage and further risks to those affected

(B) To prevent the clients from understanding the gravity of their health situation and becoming worried

(C) To prevent families and friends from becoming aware of the critical health situation of their loved ones

(D) All of the above

(49) What is hazardous material?

(A) Nonbiological material that poses no harm to living beings.

(B) Biological material that poses harm to living beings.

(C) Nonbiological material that poses some form of harm to living beings.

(D) Biological material that poses no harm to living beings.


(50) What are the three major ways to ensure safety during radiation therapy?

(A) Time, distance and shielding

(B) Handwashing, distance and shielding

(C) Disinfecting, distance and shielding

(D) Disposal, distance and time


(51) The role of nurses in ensuring client home safety includes _____.

(A) Assessing the need for home modifications

(B) Providing clients with home modification solutions

(C) Educating clients on safety issues

(D) All of the above

(52) Which of the following is a crucial factor to consider when assessing client home safety?

(A) Distance to the health care facility

(B) Slip-proof floors

(C) Number of stories

(D) All of the above

(53) How should hazardous materials be labeled?

(A) With labeling that provides specific information for identifying the nature of each hazardous material

(B) No labeling

(C) With a label that indicates danger but does not provide any specific information about the nature of the risk involved

(D) With a red label for easy recognition of danger

(54) Who should receive reports for incidents and other irregular occurrences?

(A) Clients and their family members

(B) The supervising or charge nurse and the risk management department

(C) Other health care personnel and patients

(D) All of the above


(55) Why is it important to inspect equipment for safety hazards?

(A) To ensure the equipment is functioning properly

(B) To prevent hazards, client complications and injuries

(C) To reduce the cost of equipment maintenance

(D) To identify potential legal liabilities


(56) What should nurses do when they encounter a piece of malfunctioning equipment?

(A) Dispose of the equipment immediately.

(B) Move the equipment to another client care area.

(C) Report and remove the equipment from the client care area.

(D) Attempt to fix the equipment so it can continue to be used.

(57) What are standard precautions?

(A) Preventive and infection control measures utilized to combat and inhibit the spread of specific infections.

(B) Measures taken to prevent the transfer of disease-causing organisms from one person or object to another.

(C) Infection control measures for preventing infection spread among clients, whether or not they've been diagnosed with any infection.

(D) Specialized equipment used to protect specific body areas from injury and exposure to infectious agents.

(58) What is the most effective procedure for preventing the spread of infection in health care environments?

(A) Wearing protective gloves

(B) Proper hand hygiene

(C) Disinfecting with bleach and other chemicals

(D) Using sterile equipment

(59) Which of the following is an incorrect statement about maintaining a sterile field?

(A) Wetness on the sterile field is acceptable.

(B) Staff working directly on the sterile field do not need to wear sterile masks.

(C) Nurses can turn their back to the sterile field.

(D) All of the above.


(60) What is the purpose of evaluating and monitoring the aseptic technique staff members use?

(A) To ensure that the technique is in line with generally accepted procedures

(B) To fire staff members who do not use the technique correctly

(C) To give staff members a sense of autonomy

(D) All of the above

(61) Knowledge of physiology is important in interpreting vital signs. A one-year-old baby is expected to have a _____.

(A) Higher respiratory rate compared to an adult

(B) Lower respiratory rate compared to an adult

(C) Similar respiratory rate compared to an adult

(D) None of the above


(62) A 26-year-old male presents to the emergency room. He is a known patient being managed for substance abuse and you want to counsel him on the dangers of opioid addiction. One major risk of opioid addiction is _____.

(A) Increased blood pressure

(B) Increased body temperature

(C) Depressed respiration

(D) All of the above

(63) Which of the following statements about diagnostic tests is incorrect?

(A) Materials should be by the patient's bedside before any diagnostic test.

(B) Consent is not really needed for noninvasive procedures. ✗   eg: Barium enema

(C) The procedures must be done aseptically.   Barium x-ray

(D) None of the above,   3


(64) Why should the nurse apply pressure over the site of the needle prick after a blood glucose test?

(A) Homeostasis

(B) Hemostasis ↑          ④

(C) Static equilibrium ↓

(D) Aids wound healing ✗


(65) Venipuncture is the collection of blood from a _____.

(A) Superficial vein

(B) Deep vein          5

(C) Superficial artery

(D) Deep artery

(66) Before taking any samples, what should the nurse do?

(A) Gather materials

(B) Explain the procedure

(C) Obtain consent

(D) All of the above

6    1

(67) Which of the following is not assayed for in urine?

(A) RBCs

(B) WBCs

(C) Glucose

(D) None of the above

7

(68) What kinds of cancers are closely associated with smoking?

(A) Esophageal

(B) Skin

(C) Brain

(D) All of the above

8

(69) A woman is undergoing chemotherapy for breast cancer after a mastectomy. Which of the following is not one of the potential alterations due to the chemo that you should counsel her about?

(A) Back pain

(B) Mouth sores

(C) Nausea and vomiting

9

(D) Weight changes

(70) Two main worries of invasive procedures are _____.

(A) Cost, recovery

(B) Infections, cost

10

(C) Infections, bleeding

(D) None of the above

(71) What is the first step to inserting an NG tube?

(A) Obtaining informed consent

(B) Doing a quick X-ray

(C) Inspecting the nares

(D) Hyperextending the neck

(72) What are the two types of intravenous access?

(A) Central and parenteral

(B) Parenteral and interosseous

(C) Central and peripheral          1 2

(D) All of the above


(73) Which of the following is false about urinary catheters?

(A) They can be used to void urine.

(B) They come in different sizes.          1 3

(C) Insertion is a sterile procedure.

(D) The patient should be in the prone position for catheter insertion.


(74) Which is not one of the assessments for the neurological system?

(A) Level of consciousness

(B) Mental state examination          1 4

(C) Muscle tone

(D) Muscle length

314

(75) Bell's palsy affects the facial nerve. What are the symptoms?

(A) Inability to move hands and feet

(B) Inability to make facial expressions

(C) Inability to speak

(D) All of the above

(76) Symptoms of hyperglycemia include all of the following except _____.

(A) Polydipsia

(B) Blurred vision

(C) Fatigue

(D) None of the above

(77) Some side effects of general anesthesia include _____.

(A) Persistent headaches

(C) Nausea and vomiting

(C) Drowsiness

(D) All of the above

(78) At what level can spinal anesthesia be given?

(A) L3/L4 vertebrae

(B) L2/L3 vertebrae

(C) L1/L2 vertebrae

(D) Below S1 vertebra


(79) What mechanism is not part of how the body initially deals with hypothermia?

(A) Vasodilation

(B) Vasoconstriction

(C) Shivering

(D) Increased heat rate


(80) What are some precautions to take when using the old blue light method to manage jaundice?

(A) Cover the baby's body with oil.

(B) Cover the baby's eyes.

(C) Ensure the baby is fully clothed.

(D) Ensure the light is far from the baby's skin.

(81) When assisting in invasive procedures, what is not a nurse's duty?

(A) Anticipate the next steps and make materials available at the request.

(B) Ensure all forms and documents are signed.

(C) Request an opportunity to perform an invasive procedure.

(D) Ensure informed consent is obtained.


(82) One complication associated with using ventilators is _____.

(A) Alveolar hypodistension

(B) Oxygen toxicity

(C) Life support

(D) Reduced breathing workload


(83) Why is preoxygenation done in suctioning?

(A) To maintain the airways

(B) To collapse the airways

(C) To prevent alveolar overdistension

(D) To help secretions come out more easily

(84) What are things to note about a wound?

(A) Size of the wound

(B) Discharge

(C) Color of the wound

(D) All of the above

(85) What are some specific things you should help clients avoid after surgery?

(A) PDPH

(B) Anemia

(C) Hypoglycemia

(D) Medication

(86) How do you drain the posterior bronchus of the lungs?

(A) Place the patient supine with the head of the bed elevated 45 degrees.

(B) Place the patient prone with the head of the bed elevated 45 degrees.

(C) Have the patient sit at 45 degrees.

(D) Have the patient lie down flat.

(87) What is the nurse's role in managing patients who have had an ostomy?

(A) Routine care

(B) Surgical site examination

(C) Tube inspection for patency

(D) All of the above

(88) What is an AV fistula?

(A) A connection between two arteries

(B) A connection between two veins

(C) A connection between an artery and a vein

(D) A connection between capillaries and arterioles

(89) When is the AV fistula done for dialysis?

(A) At dialysis

(B) After a week of dialysis

(C) Three months before dialysis

(D) Immediately after dialysis

(90) Which is the most abundant intracellular electrolyte?

(A) K

(B) Na

(C) Ca

(D) P

(91) A patient who has been vomiting and stooling for the past five days is at risk of _____.

(A) Hyperkalemia

(B) Hypercalcemia

(C) Hypomagnesemia

(D) Hypokalemia

(92) In which of the following conditions is hypernatremia seen?

(A) Cushing's disease

(B) Diabetes mellitus

(C) Diabetes insipidus

(D) All of the above

(93) One common cause of hypovolemia in adults is _____.

(A) Bleeding from trauma

(B) Acute diarrhea

(C) Fluid overload

(D) Gluttony

(94) Hemodynamics does not involve the _____.

(A) Study of blood flow through the vessels

(B) Study of factors responsible for the free flow of blood in vessels

(C) Studies turbulent flow of blood in vessels

(D) None of the above

(95) What is the nurse's role with a patient with arterial lines?

(A) Monitor the hemodynamic status.

(B) Check for complications.

(C) Perform other routine care.

(D) All of the above.

321

(96) Care of the patient with a pacemaker includes all of the following, except _____.

(A) Assessing the insertion site for bleeding

(B) Placing the patient on bed rest

(C) Avoiding anticoagulant medications

(D) Giving anticoagulant medications

(97) Which of the following statements is false?

(A) A telemetry technician can monitor the ECG.

(B) The nurse can monitor the ECG.

(C) Only the telemetry technician should monitor the ECG.

(D) All of the above.

(98) Which is not a pulmonary function test?

(A) Lung compliance

(B) Spirometry

(C) Forced vital capacity

(D) Chest X-ray

322

(99) Which of the following is false about a treatment plan?

(A) It includes education of the patient.

(B) It includes home care strategies.

(C) It does not include the financial implications of the treatment.

(D) It includes the financial cost of the treatment.


(100) A patient admitted and being managed for heart failure secondary to hypertensive heart disease complains of excessive and frequent urination. The patient is on the following medications: Digoxin, furosemide and lisinopril. What is the best next course of action for the nurse on duty?

(A) Stop medications immediately.

(B) Counsel the patient and allay his fears.

(C) Raise an alarm and inform the doctor on call.

(D) Pass a urinary catheter.

(101) A 60-year-old woman had a surgical procedure done which involved temporary exteriorization of the bowel loop following repair of large bowel perforation to allow for healing of the anastomosis. What was the most likely procedure done?

(A) Colostomy

(B) Colectomy

(C) Colotomy

(D) Colonoscopy

(102) A 70-year-old man was admitted on account of a cerebrovascular accident and is being managed. What is not an issue that should be anticipated by a nurse related to mobility?

(A) Speech difficulty

(B) Atelectasis

(C) Bed sores

(D) Muscle atrophy

(103) A 24-year-old high school student who was involved in a car accident is being evaluated for pain.

Arrange the following options in the correct sequence of pain ladder management.

I. "Weak" opioid or multifactorial +/- non-opioid +/-adjuvant therapy

II. Interventional treatments +/- non-opioid +/- adjuvant therapy

III. Non-opioid +/- adjuvant therapy

IV. "Strong" opioid +/- non-opioid +/- adjuvant therapy

(A) II, III, I, IV

(B) III, I, IV, I

(C) I, II, III, IV

(D) IV, III, I, II


(104) An 80-year-old woman is being managed as a case of cerebrovascular accident. Which of the following sites is an area where pressure sores associated with immobility commonly occur?

(A) Heels

(B) Elbows

(C) Knee

(D) Scapula

(105) A patient being managed for chronic insomnia is placed on sleeping medications. Which of the following is the most appropriate response in evaluating the quality of sleep?

(A) Patient slept for a longer period overnight.

(B) Patient feels refreshed after waking up.

(C) Patient tosses and turns a lot while sleeping. X

(D) Patient has several dreams while sleeping.

(106) A patient who had an exploratory laparotomy on account of bowel perforation has delayed healing of the abdominal incision site. Which of the following nutritional deficiencies is not closely related to this?

(A) Vitamin C deficiency

(B) Vitamin E deficiency

(C) Zinc deficiency

(D) Low serum protein

(107) A patient is chronically immobilized in bed due to a debilitating illness. What is an intrinsic risk factor related to pressure sores?

(A) Adequate oxygenation

(B) Elevated blood pressure

(C) Poor turning in bed

(D) Poor tissue perfusion

(108) An elderly patient was placed on total parenteral nutrition following a bowel resection for colonic cancer resection. What is the best route of venous access for this mode of nutrition?

(A) A central venous catheter

(B) A peripheral sited intravenous line with an 18-gauge cannula

(C) An intraosseous line

(D) A peripheral sited intravenous line with a 22-gauge cannula

(109) A nine-year-old boy is admitted for muscular dystrophy. During your assessment of the patient, he is able to lift his limbs from side to side but not against gravity. How would you score his muscle power on a scale of 0 to 3?

(A) 0

(B) 1

(C) 2

(D) 3

(110) As the nurse on duty during the admission of a patient, what is not a component of a detailed health assessment?

(A) Focused physical examination

(B) Detailed management plan

(C) Thorough medical history

(D) Appropriate investigation

(111) During your shift as a nurse, a patient passed away. You are counseling the relatives based on the Kübler- Ross model of grief. Which of the following is not a component of this model?

(A) Denial

(B) Acceptance     } kubler- ross model

(C) Depression

(D) Bereavement

(112) In the multidisciplinary management of a child with cerebral palsy, which of the following professionals is not necessarily needed on the team?

(A) A pediatric neurologist

(B) A neurosurgeon

(C) An occupational therapist

(D) A nutritionist

(113) A 15-year-old boy uses a single-elbow crutch due to an iatrogenic injury to the sciatic nerve during an injection in infancy. Which gait is he most likely to have?

(A) High steppage gait

(B) Waddling gait

(C) Antalgic gait

(D) Festinant gait

(114) Ray has been given a prescription for postoperative pain. But he returns before the dose is meant to be exhausted and says he lost the meds on his way home. This has happened twice. What do you think is going on?

(A) Withdrawal symptoms

(B) Drug-seeking behavior

(C) Physical dependence

(D) All of the above

(115) How do patients react when diagnosed?

(A) Some are defensive.

(B) Some are aggressive.

(C) Some mask their low self-esteem.

(D) All of the above.

(116) What is your treatment plan for a 20-year-old male patient experiencing sexual addiction?

(A) Impulse control counseling

(B) Cognitive-behavioral therapy

(C) Medications

(D) All of the above

(117) What models are used to assess a client's ability to cope with life changes?

(A) Nine model, CBT model

(B) Nagi model, social and cognitive model

(C) Coping mechanisms, client recovery model

(D) All of the above

(118) A 50-year-old man known to have attempted suicide in the past is brought to the ER in a depressed mood. His relatives say he has been having low energy and is uninterested in speaking to anyone, even his grandkids. He looks quite detached and calm at the moment. What should you watch for?

(A) Tendency to abuse medications

(B) Tendency to inflict self-harm or harm others

(C) Tendency to escape from the hospital

(D) All of the above

(119) One of your patients brought to the ER by her family has refused to speak to you. You try to ask questions, but she keeps redirecting you to a male figure who she refers to as the "head." What do you do in this situation?

(A) Quickly apologize and speak to the head.

(B) Insist on speaking to the patient.

(C) Educate the family on women's empowerment and rights.

(D) Refer the patient.

(120) Which of the following is not part of end-of-life care?

(A) Ensuring the patient is comfortable

(B) Pain medications

(C) Massage therapy

(D) Assessing discipline techniques

(121) The type of family structure where individuals can make decisions without much input from the leaders is _____.

(A) Authoritarian

(B) Laissez-faire

(C) Democratic

(D) None of the above

(122) What are Worden's tasks of mourning?

(A) Accepting the loss, coping, altering the environment, resuming a healthy life

(B) Shock and disbelief, awareness, restitution, resolution, idealization

(C) Shock, awareness of loss, conservation withdrawal, healing

(D) Denial, anger, depression, acceptance

(123) A patient has been talking excessively at his place of work. He has been wearing unusually bright colors and has been claiming he is the rightful president of the United States. He says he has the CIA working for him, even though he has never been interested in politics. His colleagues bring him to the hospital, and he keeps saying he is fine. He is just excited because it is a Tuesday. What is the likely diagnosis?

(A) Bipolar disorder

(B) Personality disorder

(C) Depressive disorder

(D) Anxiety disorder

(124) What occupational factor affecting health should a remote worker be concerned about?

(A) Commuting for long hours

(B) Sitting for long hours

(C) Standing for long hours

(D) All of the above

(125) At what stage does the patient experience increased cardiac output in Hans Selye's theory?

(A) Alarm

(B) Resistance

(C) Exhaustion

(D) A and B


(126) Your client keeps talking about his amazing wife. But you need some information about his previous medications. What do you say?

(A) "Please, can we discuss the medications now?"

(B) "Thank you so much for telling me about your wife. I am sure she is an amazing person. But can we also discuss your medications, so we can get you back home to be with her soon?"

(C) "I would prefer we discuss the medication now. Your wife is not the reason you are here."

(D) "I understand you miss your wife. But we need to get this over with the medications."

(127) All of the following are true of allergies except _____.

(A) Every human has an allergy.

(B) Signs and symptoms of allergic reactions vary per person.

(C) Allergic reactions can quickly become life-threatening.

(D) Not all allergens are life-threatening.


(128) A patient is to be given IV calcium gluconate and IV sodium bicarbonate. What is the best way to do this?

(A) Give both in quick succession.

(B) Give both slowly but immediately, one after the other.

(C) Give both within one hour.

(D) Give both one hour apart and flush the line in between both doses.


(129) Which of the following can be mixed with blood during a transfusion?

(A) Normal saline

(B) Ringer's lactate

(C) Acetaminophen

(D) None of the above

(130) Before giving blood, it is not necessary to assess _____.

(A) The religious or cultural beliefs of patients concerning transfusion

(B) If the patient has a need for a transfusion

(C) If the patient has a good intravenous line in place

(D) If the patient is sleeping


(131) Concerning ABO incompatibility, which of the following is correct?

(A) It is a form of hemoplastic blood reaction.

(B) It occurs when blood group O is transfused to blood group A.

(C) It is a hemolytic blood reaction.

(D) An agglutination reaction occurs.


(132) Which is most useful in treating severe blood transfusion reactions?

(A) Blood

(B) Supplemental oxygen

(C) Corticosteroids

(D) Antihistamines

(133) Before commencing a blood transfusion, which of the following steps is not important?

(A) Check the blood donation date.

(B) Check the blood bag details.

(C) Check pre-transfusion vital signs.

(D) Check pre-transfusion blood glucose levels.

(134) Which of these is true of peripheral lines?

(A) They are best placed in the large veins of the lower limbs.

(B) They are best placed on the hand veins.

(C) They are best placed on the dominant forearm.

(D) They are best placed on the nondominant forearm.

(135) Concerning venous access, which of the following is true?

(A) Central lines should be changed every five days.

(B) Peripheral lines are better for quick emergencies.

(C) Nurses do not need to worry about infections.

(D) Phlebitis is very uncommon with chemotherapy administration through IV lines.

338

(136) Regarding standard units of measurement for dosage calculations, which of the following is incorrect?

(A) 10 teaspoons are equal to 50 ml.

(B) 15 ml is equal to 1 tablespoon.

(C) 1 cup is equal to 15 tablespoons.

(D) 1 teaspoon is equal to 5 ml.

(137) Why is accuracy important in pharmacological measures?

(A) It affects the cost of medication.

(B) It affects the nurse's workload.

(C) It affects the patient's treatment.

(D) It affects the nurse's job performance.

(138) In drug dose calculation and administration, accuracy is very important. Why is this?

(A) Accuracy can affect the patient's treatment.

(B) Accuracy can save time for the nurse.

(C) Accuracy is a requirement for nurses' job satisfaction.

(D) Accuracy is not important in pharmacological measures.

339

(139) Which route of drug administration has 100% bioavailability?

(A) Oral route

(B) Intravenous route

(C) Transdermal route

(D) Inhalation route


(140) What is another term for total parenteral nutrition?

(A) Hyperalimentation

(B) Enteral nutrition

(C) Intravenous infusion

(D) Oral feeding


(141) How are minerals, electrolytes, vitamins, amino acids and trace elements supplied in total parenteral nutrition?

(A) Via the hyperalimentation catheter

(B) Orally

(C) Intramuscularly

(D) Through the nose

(142) What is the recommended route for administering total parenteral nutrition?

(A) Peripheral vein

(B) Oral route

(C) Central vein

(D) Intramuscular route

(143) What determines the medication dosage and strength for pain medication?

(A) The patient's age and gender

(B) The patient's medical history

(C) The patient's weight and height

(D) The level of pain and type of pain

(144) What are some examples of non-opioid analgesics?

(A) Morphine and oxycodone

(B) Aspirin and acetaminophen

(C) Fentanyl and codeine

(D) Methadone and hydromorphone

(145) What are some examples of nonpharmacological pain management techniques?

(A) Heat therapy, cold therapy and massage

(B) Antibiotics, corticosteroids and diuretics

(C) Chemotherapy, radiation therapy and surgery

(D) Cardiac catheterization, angioplasty and bypass surgery


(146) What should health care providers do when assessing pain in patients who are difficult to communicate with?

(A) Disregard their pain.

(B) Assume they have no pain.

(C) Use pain scales and observation.

(D) Rely solely on patient self-reports.


(147) What is the role of patient education in pain management?

(A) To discourage patients from seeking pain relief

(B) To promote self-management and adherence to the pain management plan

(C) To minimize patient involvement in pain management

(D) To discourage communication about pain with health care providers

(148) What is the rationale for using upper limbs for intravenous therapy?

(A) Lower-limb phlebitis can be avoided.

(B) Upper limbs have larger veins.

(C) It is easier to access veins in upper limbs.

(D) Upper limbs are less prone to infections.


(149) Who can care for central lines and venous access devices in intravenous therapy?

(A) Physician

(B) Nursing assistant

(C) RN

(D) Physical therapist

(150) What are reliable sources for nurses to obtain information about a patient's medications?

(A) Patient's family members ✗

(B) Social media

(C) Nurse's intuition

(D) Nurse's drug handbook, nursing textbook, formulary, pharmacist and trustworthy internet resources

# Test 2: Answers and Explanations

**(1) (B) Uniform Anatomical Gift Act.**

This act allows living clients to donate their body parts in the US. It allows relatives of a deceased individual to decide to donate an organ if the individual did not decide while alive. It also includes several regulations that prevent the sale or trafficking of human body parts.

**(2) (A) Value history.**

This document describes the beliefs, opinions and principles of the client. Although it is not a legal document, it is useful in determining some decisions on how a patient is handled and how the beliefs that they hold affect their treatment and care.

**(3) (A) Turning the stroke patient.**

Turning the stroke patient does not require high professional judgment since the patient is stable. But resuscitating the 25-year-old man will require a general assessment of his condition, fluid status and mental health status, which would be more appropriate for an RN to do.

(4) (D) None of the above.

Nursing case management involves developing, implementing and evaluating patient health care plans. But beyond this, it is an effective method of delivering nursing care. It typically involves managing and coordinating care, identifying and effectively utilizing resources, planning referrals and connecting clients to services based on need.

(5) (D) All of the above.

The plan developed for each patient must be individualized based on the patient's condition and need. The plan must consider several factors about the client, such as the diagnosis, ability to take care of oneself, the currently prescribed treatment, actual and potential problems. The plan must always remain up to date based on the current needs of the client.

(6) (B) HIPAA.

HIPAA protects the client's personal information, e.g., the name, date of birth, social security number, diagnosis and treatment. This act ensures that only those involved in the management or care of the patient have access to health information.

(7) (C) Providing inaccurate information about their health status.

Client responsibilities include treating health care workers with respect, paying medical bills and resolving other financial obligations as soon as possible, reporting changes that are unexpected in their condition to health care professionals, providing accurate information about their health, following rules and regulations given upon admission and being responsible for their behavior.

(8) (D) Rejecting or accepting interventions on behalf of the patient.

The goal of advocacy is to speak on behalf of patients and defend their rights and interests at all times. Advocacy can be in different forms. It might involve extensive education and sensitization of the patient and client families. It also involves explaining diagnoses, tests or examination findings. However, it is not the place of the nurse to accept or reject an intervention on behalf of a patient. Let patients and their families decide what they want.

(9) (C) Assess the client.

The first step is to assess the client's needs and whether the nursing staff and other health care professionals can adequately meet the need.

(10) (D) All of the above.

To triage effectively, a nurse must be organized and composed. A nurse must be able to diagnose conditions appropriately and have a high suspicion index. A nurse must be an excellent time manager to ensure that the right medications are given at the right time in the right doses. Any RN must also be an expert manager of people to get them to work together as a team to achieve quality health care delivery.

(11) (D) All of the above.

A nurse should be able to communicate effectively with others so that work is done at the right time. A nurse should also plan work systematically, making room for changes in the status or condition of clients and priorities. The health care setting is usually very busy, and if care is not taken, less urgent tasks can get in the way of urgent tasks. Therefore, it is the responsibility of a nurse to decline such tasks when there are other urgent tasks to perform.

(12) (B) Sentinel event.

A sentinel event refers to an incident or accident that led to or could potentially cause harm to a client. In this question, the sentinel event was the transfusion of the two pints of blood, which led to a severe transfusion reaction.

(13) (B) Outcome measures.

Outcome measures focus on the outcomes of care. They focus on the results that are obtained as a result of health care delivered to a client. They include MRSA infection rates, lengths of stay, the effectiveness of fall prevention and morbidity rates.

(14) (D) All of the above.

Nurses collaborate with other members of the health care team to deliver quality health care. Nurses must maintain high professionalism, good interpersonal and communication skills and sound judgment when interacting with other health care professionals.

(15) (D) All of the above.

Nurses can serve as patient advocates at interdisciplinary conferences, raising issues pertinent to client care. They can also resolve potential conflict issues and areas of misunderstanding with other professionals. Interdisciplinary conferences are necessary for the holistic management of patients. They provide the opportunity to contribute to client care and learn and observe from the perspective of other health care professionals.

(16) (D) Frustration.

At this point, the people involved in the conflict feel like their needs, whatever they are, are being sidelined. It might be a need for respect, consideration of working hours, a bonus or raise or a client feeling neglected.

(17) (B) Individuals respond to the frustrations and conclusions they have arrived at.

The action state of conflict is when individuals act on the frustrations and conclusions they have come to. At this point, the action taken differs. For some, the action taken might be lashing out in anger or physical assault. Others might withdraw and avoid the person involved.

(18) (A) Random blood glucose.

The most important investigation for this client is a random blood glucose check since he is a known Type I DM. He is most likely suffering from hypoglycemia secondary to insulin overdose or administration without eating. Fasting blood glucose, urine tests and CBC can also be useful later on. But at the moment, the most important test is random blood glucose.

(19) (C) As often as needed.

Health care plans should be revised as often as needed whenever there is a change in a patient's condition. Patients are always in a dynamic state. The plan of care must be adjusted to their needs. When there is an improvement, the plan of care should be updated, and if otherwise, the plan of care should be adjusted to suit the new state.

(20) (B) Ethical dilemmas cannot be avoided in nursing care.

As nurses practice the delivery of care, ethical dilemmas will definitely arise because there are different types of patients, conditions and cases that will be encountered. The nurse must be grounded in the ethics of the profession to make the right decisions.

(21) (D) A and B.

The purpose of the code of ethics is to provide a framework for decision-making and to set responsibility reminders for nurses.

(22) (B) The code of ethics must be revised.

The code of ethics is revised from time to time to cover development in the world. This includes changes in technology, the community and expanding nursing practice into advanced practice roles, research, education, health policy and administration.

(23) (D) 11/12/20 0830 hrs. IV acetaminophen 900 mg STAT given. The patient reports pain as 5/10.

The right way to input information is the date, time, the drug and the correct route of administration, the dose, the frequency and the assessment of the patient.

(24) (B) "I am sorry, I cannot allow you to see that."

Let her know that you must keep such information private. HIPAA protects the client's personal information, e.g., the name, date of birth, social security number, diagnosis and treatment. This act ensures that only those involved in the management or care of the patient have access to health care information.

(25) (D) "I will get you a copy from the records office."

According to the Patient's Bill of Rights, patients have the right to review their medical records and request an amendment of any inaccurate information.

(26) (B) 4 times daily.

PRN means as often as needed. Three times daily is TDS, and BD is twice daily. Drugs are usually administered as regularly as needed or as prescribed. "QDS" or "qid" is an abbreviation for the Latin term "quater in die", which translates to "four times a day".

(27) (D) Not evaluating the patient for stroke.

A transient ischemic attack is a risk factor for stroke, and not evaluating a TIA patient for stroke would be considered negligence.

(28) (C) A five-year-old boy whose weight for his age is below normal.

This child might need a targeted nutritional assessment because his weight for his age is already below normal. Target screening can be done when some people show strong tendencies, signs or symptoms of a particular condition or disease. This target screening is also done when a client is at risk of a certain ailment or there is a need to rule out a possible condition.

(29) (A) Nonjudgmental.

Nurses should be open, trusting and nonjudgmental. No matter the condition, they should be open to understanding the client's perspective, even if what the person is saying is not correct from a professional stance.

(30) (D) Exercise.

High-risk behaviors are actions that significantly increase the likelihood of harm, disease or death. Most of these behaviors are modifiable behaviors that are based on choice. They can include diet, a sedentary lifestyle, violence and drug abuse.

(31) (D) 4.

Physical readiness involves the measure of ability, the complexity of the task, the effect of the environment, the health status of the individual and even gender. Mental readiness deals more with the cognitive and psychological aspects of readiness. Experiential readiness deals with the levels of aspiration, coping mechanisms used in the past, the locus of control orientation and self-efficacy. Knowledge readiness refers to the current level of knowledge of the learner, the level of capacity to learn and the preferred style of learning of the individual.

(32) (B) Literacy.

Literacy helps learning. Illiteracy is a barrier to learning. Cultural and spiritual beliefs can be barriers to learning. Language can also be a limitation if an interpreter is not made available. When clients are in pain, they cannot concentrate on whatever is being communicated to them. Hence learning is hindered.

(33) (B) Moderately distressed, needs moderate resuscitation.

Each parameter in the APGAR score is assessed as 0, 1 or 2, and the total is added up to 10. If a child is scored less than 4, then the child is in severe distress and will need urgent intensive care and resuscitation. A score of 4–6 is moderately distressed and requires moderate attention and resuscitation. Neonates who score 7 and above are in excellent condition.

(34) (D) Mastering toilet training.

Toddlers are at Erikson's second stage of development, autonomy vs. shame and doubt. At this stage, children are focused on the development of self-control. At this stage they are expected to master toilet training.

(35) (B) Decreased self-consciousness.

WHO defines adolescence as between 10–19 years. There is increased identity definition at this stage of development. At this stage you should expect to see attraction toward the opposite sex, increased self-consciousness and seeking peer group acceptance.

(36) (D) A and B.

This is the final stage of psychosocial development and it is seen in the elderly. It is called the integrity vs. despair stage, and people at this point usually look retrospectively at the influence of the choices they made earlier in life. They experience a gradual decline in physical function and musculature and some of the changes that are associated with aging in their body systems.

(37) (D) Placenta separation.

Active management of the third stage of labor involves administering 10 IU of oxytocin a minute after delivery to help the uterus contract, ensuring that the entire placenta is delivered through controlled cord traction and uterine massage. Placenta separation occurs on its own, and only after it has occurred can the placenta be delivered through controlled cord traction.

(38) (B) Fetal heart Doppler.

The fetal heart Doppler is a device that is used to monitor the heartbeat of the fetus in the uterus. Using this device creates a simulation of the fetal heartbeat; some devices display the value per minute. The sounds can also be heard and counted over a minute.

(39) (D) Elevated fetal heart rate.

Elevated fetal heart rate can be a strong indicator of fetal distress. Heart rates exceeding 160 bpm are considered elevated and demand urgent medical attention. Decreased fetal movement is more useful before labor and is usually assessed through a fetal kick chart.

(40) (B) Postpartum hemorrhage.

Postpartum hemorrhage is defined as blood loss greater than 500 ml for SVD or greater than 1000 ml after a cesarean section. It is also defined as any volume of blood loss that results in hemodynamic instability of the patient after delivery.

(41) (C) Comfort and safety.

The client care environment refers to the physical and social setting in which nursing care is provided. Assessing the client care environment involves considering factors such as safety, comfort, privacy and cultural sensitivity. Safety is a priority, and nurses should ensure that environments where patients are to be attended to are continually kept safe from threats and potential hazards.

(42) (A) Privacy is not a factor of concern when assessing the client care environment.

The client care environment must also be assessed for physical and emotional comfortability. One component of emotional comfort is privacy.

(43) (D) All of the above.

Some things that can be done to promote staff safety include providing education and training, providing PPE, creating a safe and ideal work environment and encouraging staff communication.

(44) (B) Every 2 hours.

Patients who cannot change their positions by themselves should be turned every two hours while being kept in a position that will cause no harm and bring minimal stress to muscle groups. The nurses should ensure this is done to prevent the formation of bed sores.

(45) (D) A patient who cannot communicate in English.

A patient who needs help communicating in English or the official language of communication in the client care environment is highly prone to identification errors. To avoid this, such patients have a right to an interpreter so they can understand all that is communicated to them.

(46) (C) Irrespective of where they occur and who is affected.

RNs should be trained to handle all kinds of emergencies, including those within or outside their medical facilities' confines and those within or outside their communities. Nurses' response to the crisis is not based on who is affected, nor is it based on color, race or any other form of bias.

(47) (B) Ambulatory clients.

Ambulatory clients who require little or no assistance should be the first to be discharged after they have been treated, given prescriptions and received other necessary instructions. Unstable patients are high-priority clients and are, therefore, not candidates for discharge.

(48) (A) To prevent sabotage and further risks to those affected.

RNs should be able to use intuition to discern and plan ahead for the most effective ways to communicate during emergencies to avoid sabotage and additional risks that could come to patients due to leaked information.

(49) (C) Nonbiological material that poses some form of harm to living beings.

Hazardous materials are defined as nonbiological materials that pose some form of harm to human beings, animals and other living components of the environment. Hazardous materials can be anything ranging from harmful chemicals and radiation to soiled and used equipment like needles that could become potential sources of infection.

(50) (A) Time, distance and shielding.

Nurses and technicians should ensure clients have the most minimal exposure to radiation by minimizing exposure time, ensuring safe distance and using shielding.

(51) (D) All of the above.

Nurses, alongside other health care staff, work together to assess clients' homes, identify safety concerns, proffer solutions or modifications and educate on safety issues to provide an enabling home environment for clients.

(52) (B) Slip-proof floors.

Slip-proof floors are crucial to improving the well-being of patients and adjusting their lifestyles to new health conditions. Other factors, such as distance to the health care facility, are irrelevant to determining client safety.

(53) (A) With labeling that provides specific information for identifying the nature of each hazardous material.

Hazardous materials should be properly labeled so that even the layman can identify the risk. There should, however, also be labeling that provides specific information for identifying the nature of each hazardous material.

(54) (B) The supervising or charge nurse and the risk management department.

Reports should go to the health care facility's supervising or charge nurse and the risk management department.

(55) (B) To prevent hazards, client complications and injuries.

Inspecting equipment before use is crucial for preventing hazards, client complications and injuries to health care workers.

(56) (C) Report and remove the equipment from the client care area.

Unsafe and malfunctioning equipment should be reported and moved from the client care area to ensure optimal safety. Faulty equipment should only be discarded if it has been designated irredeemable by a professional technician.

(57) (C) Infection control measures for preventing infection spread among clients, whether or not they've been diagnosed with any infection.

Standard precautions are the minimum infection prevention practices that should be used in health care settings for all patients. They are designed to reduce the risk of transmission of microorganisms from recognized and unrecognized infection sources.

(58) (B) Proper hand hygiene.

Proper hand hygiene, such as washing with mild soap and water, disinfecting when necessary and wearing protective gloves, prevents thousands of infections from spreading in health care environments.

(59) (D) All of the above.

Only sterile items should be placed on the sterile field. Nurses should never have a sterile field below the waist level. They should not lean over or ever turn their backs to the sterile field. Coughing or sneezing over the sterile field contaminates it. All staff in or around a sterile field should wear gowns and gloves. Those working directly on the sterile field should use sterile masks.

(60) (A) To ensure that the technique is in line with generally accepted procedures.

RNs should evaluate and monitor the staff members when carrying out aseptic techniques to ascertain competency and adherence to procedures.

(61) (A) Higher respiratory rate compared to an adult.

A one-year-old baby has a smaller lung volume compared to an adult and therefore has to breathe faster to exchange gases. Babies also metabolize faster, so they need to exchange waste products faster than adults.

(62) (C) Depressed respiration.

Some of the other signs of opioid intoxication include euphoria, reduced anxiety, hypotension from hypovolemia, miosis and altered regulation of body temperature.

(63) (B) Consent is not really needed for noninvasive procedures.

The testing kits and equipment should be by the patient's bedside to start any diagnostic test. The nurse should do a brief introduction of the whole process. The patient must give consent to the test before proceeding. Proper handwashing before and after the test is essential to keep the process aseptic.

(64) (B) Hemostasis.

The nurse presses the puncture site with sterile gauze until the blood stops flowing. Applying pressure this way reduces the flow of blood to that vessel and also allows for clotting factors to quickly get to work.

(65) (A) Superficial vein.

Blood collection is from a superficial vein, usually in the upper limb. This is because superficial veins are close to the skin and are easily accessible.

(66) (D) All of the above.

The nurse should first explain the process to the patient and obtain consent. Then the nurse can gather materials, the skin is cleaned with an alcohol swab, and the arm is tied with a tourniquet to make the veins more visible. A cannula is introduced into the vein slowly and blood is collected into a bottle.

(67) (D) None of the above.

Proteins, blood cells, glucose and other chemicals are assayed in the urine. Urine is routinely collected for urinary tract infections, sexually transmitted infections and renal diseases.

(68) (A) Esophageal.

Patients exposed to cigarette smoke are at risk of lung, esophageal and oral cancers. Patients with a family history of cancer are at risk. Patients whose occupation exposes them to ultraviolet radiation are predisposed to skin cancers.

(69) (A) Back pain.

The major alterations that happen secondary to chemotherapy include weight changes, nausea and vomiting, mouth sores, anemia, sleep difficulty, skin and nail changes, loss of appetite, easy bruising and bleeding and infections.

(70) (C) Infections, bleeding.

Some noninvasive procedures are costlier than invasive procedures. However, invasive procedures always have concerns around infections because the skin barrier is breached and bleeding. Once infections and bleeding are not present, recovery is usually swift.

(71) (A) Obtaining informed consent.

Consent must always be obtained before beginning any procedure.

(72) (C) Central and peripheral.

There are two ways to secure intravenous access—central and peripheral access. A peripheral intravenous line is used for short-term purposes like administering fluids, chemotherapy and electrolytes. Central venous access is for more long-term purposes.

(73) (D) The patient should be in the prone position for catheter insertion.

This is false. To insert a urinary catheter, the patient should be in the supine position for insertion. The nurse should expose the patient's thighs and pelvic region. The patient separates the thighs to give access to the perineal area. The catheter is inserted into the urethral meatus and advanced above the point when urine is seen in the catheter. The nurse should inflate the catheter to secure it in the urethra. The catheter is then connected to the urine bag and attached to the patient's leg.

(74) (D) Muscle length.

Assessing the neurological system requires appropriately assessing the cranial nerves, level of consciousness, muscle tone and mental status. A patient's level of consciousness is set as oriented to time, place and person. A patient isn't fully conscious if he or she doesn't know the time of the day, is confused about the date and doesn't know where he or she is.

(75) (B) Inability to make facial expressions.

The facial nerve is assessed for the ability to feel sensory impulses of the face and move the muscles of the face to make facial expressions.

(76) (D) None of the above.

Hyperglycemia can present with polydipsia, urinary frequency, blurred vision, dehydration and fatigue.

(77) (D) All of the above.

General anesthesia makes the client completely unconscious. Patients are intubated and placed on mechanical ventilation throughout the procedure. It is laborious and requires continuous monitoring. It is also essential to monitor the amount of anesthetic given as it can have dangerous side effects.

(78) (A) L3/L4 vertebrae.

In spinal anesthesia, where an anesthetic is injected into the subarachnoid space, the sites for administration are either between the L3/L4 or the L4/L5 vertebrae.

(79) (A) Vasodilation.

In hypothermia, the body's temperature falls lower than normal and the body tries to generate heat by shivering and conserve heat by vasoconstriction, not vasodilation.

(80) (B) Cover the baby's eyes.

The baby's eyes must be covered to prevent possible retinal damage. However, the baby cannot be fully clothed during phototherapy with lights, or the radiation will not penetrate the skin. The light should be close to the baby's skin, typically about 10 cm or as stated by the manufacturer.

(81) (C) Request an opportunity to perform the invasive procedure.

Physicians and licensed practitioners do most invasive procedures. But nurses can assist them, so it is necessary to know about these procedures, the steps and the complications. Some invasive procedures include central venous lines, needle biopsies, spinal taps and intubations.

(82) (B) Oxygen toxicity.

Oxygen toxicity is another complication to look out for. The blood is being saturated continually by air containing oxygen under high pressure. Thus, there is a tendency for the blood to be oversaturated with oxygen.

(83) (A) To maintain the airways.

Oxygen is administered before suctioning to maintain the airways during suctioning. Preoxygenation involves increasing inspired oxygen just before suctioning. It has been suggested that preoxygenation can prevent some of the side effects of endotracheal suctioning, for instance, hypoxemia.

(84) (D) All of the above.

The wound area is inspected regularly. The color, size, presence of pus, surrounding structures and odor of the pus are examined. The drainage of the wound can be bloody, serous, serosanguinous and purulent.

(85) (A) PDPH.

Patients with spinal or epidural anesthesia should not raise their heads for a few hours after the procedure to prevent postdural puncture headaches (PDPHs). PDPH occurs as a result of the leakage of cerebrospinal fluid through the hole created by the needle when anesthesia is administered. The reduction in CSF volume causes a stretch of the cranial nerves, which presents as a headache. The headache is usually positional and frontal.

(86) (B) Place the patient prone, with the head of the bed elevated 45 degrees.

The patient is prone and the bed is elevated to a 45-degree position. This drains respiratory secretions from the posterior bronchus.

(87) (D) All of the above.

The surgical wound site is examined as part of care for ostomies. Nurses maintain the tubes' patency and change them as needed. For tracheostomies, the nurse monitors the respiratory secretions' input and output.

(88) (C) A connection between an artery and a vein.

An AV is a connection between an artery and a vein.

(89) (C) Three months before dialysis.

An AV is a connection between an artery and vein and is done three months before the dialysis to allow for maturity.

(90) (A) K.

Potassium (K) is the most abundant intracellular electrolyte. Sodium (Na) is the most abundant extracellular electrolyte. Calcium (Ca) is both intracellular and extracellular, but predominantly intracellular. Phosphorus (P) is mostly deposited in bone, but also has some intracellular and extracellular qualities.

(91) (D) Hypokalemia.

Hypokalemia is the reduction in the potassium levels in the blood below the usual standard. Hypokalemia can be a result of diarrhea, vomiting and diaphoresis. Hypokalemia is characterized by muscle weakness, tingling, numbness, constipation and even cardiac arrest.

(92) (C) Diabetes insipidus.

In diabetes insipidus, there is a loss of large volumes of water, which results in a depleted fluid volume and an increase in osmotic concentration, which can result in hypernatremia.

(93) (A) Bleeding from trauma.

Hypovolemia is a reduction in the fluid in the blood. Hypovolemia may occur as a result of bleeding, vomiting and diarrhea, but the most common cause is bleeding from trauma. Fluid overload does not cause hypovolemia. Gluttony only results in hypovolemia if there is associated vomiting and diarrhea, which is very severe.

(94) (D) None of the above.

Hemodynamics is the study of how blood flows through the blood vessels.

(95) (D) All of the above.

Nurses should know the complications, such as infections, trauma, hematomas and scar tissue formation. Nurses monitor the hemodynamic status of patients with arterial lines. They also anticipate the complications and manage accordingly.

(96) (D) Giving anticoagulant medications.

For a patient with a pacemaker, the insertion site of the pacemaker should be assessed for bleeding and infections. The nurse should maintain bed rest and avoid giving the patient heparin or aspirin, which are anticoagulants.

(97) (C) Only the telemetry technician should monitor the ECG.

Telemetry involves continuously monitoring and recording ECG strips. Telemetry is mostly done by a telemetry technician, but nurses can monitor telemetry too.

(98) (D) Chest X-ray.

Patients with impaired ventilation/oxygenation should be assessed with pulmonary function tests like pulse oximetry, spirometry, lung compliance and forced vital capacity. A chest X-ray, however, is not a pulmonary function test, even though it can be used to visualize the lungs and pleural space.

(99) (C) It does not include the financial implications of the treatment.

This is false. As part of the treatment plan, the patient should be told about the treatment procedures and the financial cost of each treatment. Nurses should teach patients about home care strategies for their illnesses. The patients should receive a follow-up schedule as part of the treatment plan.

(100) (B) Counsel the patient and allay his fears.

The best next course of action is to counsel and allay the patient's fear, as excessive and frequent urination is a known side effect of medications used to treat heart failure and hypertensive heart disease.

(101) (A) Colostomy.

A colostomy is a surgical procedure done to establish an artificial connection between the lumen of the colon and the skin, which has varying indications. The indication in this case is to rest the repair site of the perforated bowel. It is important to be aware of common surgical procedures, indications and effects on management.

(102) (A) Speech difficulty.

Speech difficulty is not a primary issue related to mobility. It is, however, related to the primary pathology. Other answer options are systemic complications of prolonged immobility and should be anticipated and prevented.

(103) (B) III, I, IV, I.

Based on the WHO analgesic ladder, pain management is usually started with the least non-opioids to opioids and, finally, other interventional treatments to manage severe pain.

(104) (C) Knee.

Pressure sores commonly occur on bony prominences, which are in prolonged contact with the bed. Due to immobility, patients usually lie decubitus in bed; hence the knees are usually facing upward and are rarely in contact with the bed.

(105) (B) Patient feels refreshed after waking up.

Feeling refreshed after waking up is the best response to assess the quality of sleep, as the duration of sleep and other parameters do not fully reflect improvement in insomnia management.

(106) (B) Vitamin E deficiency.

Vitamin E deficiency is not closely related to delayed wound healing. Deficiencies in Vitamin C, A, zinc, copper and low serum protein are associated with poor wound healing postoperatively as they are required for collagen formation.

(107) (D) Poor tissue perfusion.

Poor tissue perfusion is an intrinsic factor related to pressure sores. Adequate oxygenation prevents pressure sores. Elevated blood pressure has little effect on pressure sores. Poor turning in bed is an extrinsic factor related to pressure sores.

(108) (A) A central venous catheter.

A central venous catheter is the best route for administration of TPN as it lasts longer, does not get blocked easily and nutrients enter the bloodstream faster, unlike the other routes.

(109) (C) 2.

Muscle power is graded on a scale of 0 to 5.

0 – No movement at all.
1 – Flicker of movement.
2 – Cannot move against gravity but can move from side to side.  —
3 – Can move against gravity but not resistance.  —
4 – Can move against gravity and mild to moderate resistance.
5 – Full power.

(110) (A) Focused physical examination.

During a detailed health assessment of a patient, a complete physical examination should be done rather than a focused physical examination.

(111) (D) Bereavement.

The Kübler-Ross model of grief includes the following stages: Denial is when the person refuses to accept the loss that has occurred. Anger can be directed at oneself, the family, friends or the world. Bargaining involves bargaining with a higher power. Depression is felt when the person begins to really feel the loss. Acceptance is living with the new reality that the loved one is truly gone. Bereavement is not a component of the model.

(112) (B) A neurosurgeon.

A neurosurgeon is not necessarily needed in the management of cerebral palsy. Professionals needed include a pediatric neurologist, pediatric nurse, occupational therapist, physiotherapist, nutritionist, speech therapist, ENT surgeon and orthopedic surgeon.

(113) (A) High steppage gait.

High steppage gait is usually seen in patients with sciatic nerve injury leading to foot drop, hence the need for high leg clearance during walking. Waddling gait is seen in developmental dysplasia of the hip. Antalgic is seen in pain of limb infection, and Festinant gait is usually seen in Parkinson's disease.

(114) (B) Drug-seeking behavior.

Ray is exhibiting drug-seeking behavior. Other manifestations of drug-seeking behavior include claiming medications have been exhausted, falsifying prescriptions or always having an ailment that requires medication.

(115) (D) All of the above.

When clients are diagnosed, the nurse needs to observe them and their reactions. Some clients might be defensive, and others might feel ashamed. Some clients might immediately admit their problem and then seek a way out. Others might blame others and rationalize their behavior. Some clients might present with low self-esteem masked with a buoyant personality or aggression.

(116) (D) All of the above.

Sexual addiction is a non-substance-related addiction. For clients in this category, impulse control counseling and therapy would be useful. Cognitive-behavioral therapy and drug therapy can also be beneficial in addressing these disorders.

(117) (B) Nagi model, social and cognitive model.

Social and cognitive models emphasize that clients should remain as independent as possible. They can still control their reactions to the environment, and as such, the individual should be allowed to gain mastery over the situation, not be pitied or looked down upon. The Nagi model emphasizes that disability is a function of the social environment's expectations and the client's inability to meet them.

(118) (B) Tendency to inflict self-harm or harm others.

Some of the risk factors for self-harm and violence to others include a history of depression, a history of self-harm, a history of depression, age greater than 45 years, past suicide attempts, non-heterosexual orientations and joblessness.

(119) (A) Quickly apologize and speak to the head.

Nurses must always ensure they allow for their clients' cultural practices and beliefs when providing care. This determines if the care will be received or rejected many times. No matter how different a culture might be, a nurse must respect it as long as it does not harm the client or other clients in the hospital.

(120) (D) Assessing discipline techniques.

End-of-life care should be adequately provided for clients who need it. This care might include proper hygiene, ensuring the patient is comfortable and providing privacy. It might include proper turning and positioning of the patient at regular intervals. It can also include massage, therapy and any other treatment the client needs.

(121) (B) Laissez-faire.

Some families operate in an authoritarian structure where the leader makes all the decisions without room for deliberation among family members. Others run a democratic structure where all family members can deliberate on matters and decisions to be made. Some other families run a laissez-faire leadership where individuals within the family unit are left to make their own decisions while the leaders support and provide the needed resources.

(122) (A) Accepting the loss, coping, altering the environment, resuming a healthy life.

Worden's four tasks of mourning include accepting the loss, coping with the loss, altering the environment to cope with the loss and resuming a healthy life.

(123) (A) Bipolar disorder.

Bipolar disorder presents with episodes of manic and hypomanic depression occurring at intervals. Signs and symptoms include elevated mood, irritability, depressed mood, restlessness, loss of inhibition, increased sexual drive, loss of sleep and grandiose delusion.

(124) (B) Sitting for long hours.

Sitting for long hours at a stretch can be a risk factor for cardiovascular diseases. It can be an indication of a sedentary lifestyle, which is also a risk factor for cardiovascular illnesses and obesity. It can also lead to diabetes, increased cholesterol, DVT and dementia.

(125) (D) A and B.

There is increased cardiac output in both stages for different reasons. In the alarm stage, these manifestations aim to prepare the patient to flee. The resistance stage is marked by increased cardiac output and a maintained respiratory rate and blood pressure increase. Here, the body is trying to deal with the effects of stress.

(126) (B) "Thank you so much for telling me about your wife. I am sure she is an amazing person. But can we also discuss your medications, so we can get you back home to be with her soon?"

This is called focusing. A nurse must be able to focus the discussion on the important issues at hand, even when the client wants to divert to other things not as important or pertinent at the moment.

(127) (A) Every human has an allergy.

It is not established that all human beings have allergies; however, signs and symptoms of allergic reactions may vary per person and per exposure. Some reactions can also be life-threatening.

(128) (D) Give both one hour apart and flush the line in between both doses.

This is the most appropriate way to give such a combination, as giving them in quick succession can cause a chemical reaction that can damage the vein or cause a reaction. This is why a good knowledge of chemistry and pharmacology is important in nursing practice to identify such issues.

(129) (D) None of the above.

Mixing any substance with blood during a transfusion is not advisable to prevent lysing blood components or causing a transfusion reaction. Even if the substance is not known to cause a reaction, it should not be mixed with blood.

(130) (D) If the patient is sleeping.

Instead of assessing if the patient is asleep, it is better to assess the vital signs and sensorium of the patient. The religious or cultural beliefs of patients are very important as some people with religious beliefs do not accept blood transfusions; an example is Jehovah's Witnesses.

(131) (C) It is a hemolytic blood reaction.

It is a hemolytic agglutination reaction that occurs with the transfusion of mismatched blood types.

(132) (B) Supplemental oxygen.

There may be an imminent cardiorespiratory failure in severe blood transfusion reactions, and the patient may require supplemental oxygen and pharmaceuticals. Corticosteroids and antihistamines are useful in mild to moderate reactions. Blood is not needed for this emergency.

(133) (D) Check pre-transfusion blood glucose levels.

It is very important to check the blood donation date as this will help to know how fresh the blood is, as some conditions warrant fresh whole blood. Also, ensuring the blood bag details are correct will help prevent blood transfusion reactions due to clerical errors. Pre-transfusion vital signs help to know when the patient reacts to the blood. Blood glucose levels do not affect blood transfusion.

(134) (D) They are best placed on the nondominant forearm.

Peripheral venous catheters are best placed on the nondominant forearm to enable the patient to use the dominant limb for other activities. Lower extremities are avoided because of attendant complications of phlebitis.

(135) (B) Peripheral lines are better for quick emergencies

Because of the level of expertise needed to secure central venous access, it is less suitable for emergencies. Central lines should be changed every 48 hours. Infections should be a concern with venous lines. Chemotherapy is notable for cellular damage.

(136) (C) 1 cup is equal to 15 tablespoons.

One cup is equal to 15 tablespoons. Also, 1 teaspoon equals 5 ml, so 10 teaspoons equal 50 ml.

(137) (C) It affects the patient's treatment.

It affects the patient's treatment. Accuracy in dosage, routes and concentration of medications is important to ensure proper patient treatment. If the dosage is less than what is needed, then the effect of the drug will not be as potent as it should be. If the dosage is higher, then toxicity might set in.

(138) (A) Accuracy can affect the patient's treatment.

Accuracy in pharmacological measures, such as medication dosage calculations, is critical to ensure that patients receive the correct amount of medication their health care provider prescribes. Incorrect dosages can have serious consequences, including ineffective treatment or adverse effects on the patient's health.

T- 5
Tan - 15

(139) (B) Intravenous route.

All the medication administered into the veins will reach the target organs; hence only the intravenous route has 100% bioavailability.

(140) (A) Hyperalimentation.

Total parenteral nutrition, known as hyperalimentation, is administered through a more prominent vein, such as the subclavian vein. Hyperalimentation can meet all dietary requirements, with feedings containing minerals, electrolytes, vitamins, amino acids and trace elements supplied via the hyperalimentation catheter, which the physician surgically implants.

(141) (A) Via the hyperalimentation catheter.

Minerals, electrolytes, vitamins, amino acids and trace elements are supplied via the hyperalimentation catheter, which is surgically implanted.

(142) (C) Central vein.

The recommended route for administering total parenteral nutrition is through the central vein. Parenteral nutrition cannot be given via peripheral veins because of the increased risk of thrombophlebitis when administered peripherally. The central line also allows a large quantity of nutrients to be given over a shorter period of time.

(143) (D) The level of pain and type of pain.

The level of pain and type of pain are what will determine the medication dosage and strength of the pain medication to be administered.


(144) (B) Aspirin and acetaminophen.

Aspirin and acetaminophen are examples of non-opioid analgesics. The rest of the options, morphine and oxycodone, fentanyl and codeine and methadone and hydromorphone, are examples of opioid analgesics.


(145) (A) Heat therapy, cold therapy and massage.

Heat therapy, cold therapy and massage are examples of nonpharmacological pain management techniques.


(146) (C) Use pain scales and observation.

With the use of pain scales and observation, a subjective assessment can be made of the patient's pain level.


(147) (B) To promote self-management and adherence to the pain management plan.

Patient education promotes self-management and adherence to the pain management plan.

(148) (A) Lower-limb phlebitis can be avoided

Upper limbs are used wherever possible to avoid lower-limb phlebitis and emboli. DVT is very common with lower limb veins, and it should be avoided at all costs. Upper limb veins can also sometimes be more accessible than lower limb veins. They are also easy for cannula placement and infusion drips.

(149) (C) RN.

RNs are responsible for caring for central lines and venous access devices in intravenous therapy.

(150) (D) Nurses' drug handbook, nursing textbook, formulary, pharmacist and trustworthy internet resources.

The nurses' drug handbook, a nursing textbook, a formulary, a pharmacist and trustworthy internet resources are reliable sources that nurses can access and obtain information about a patient's medications.

# Test 3 Questions

(1) Greg was admitted to a hospital after an automobile accident in which he lost a lot of blood. His hematocrit was very low, and a transfusion was recommended. However, he declined to receive blood via transfusion for personal reasons. What did Greg exercise here?

(A) Right to privacy

(B) Self-determination act

(C) Health care proxy

(D) Uniform Anatomical Gift Act

(2) Which of the following is not true about delegation?

(A) It means the transfer of responsibility.

(B) The nurse delegating retains no responsibility for the outcome of the delegated task.

(C) The nurse delegating still retains responsibility for the outcome of the delegated task.

(D) All of the above.

(3) What is the basis of selecting the right person for a task?

(A) Skills and knowledge

(B) Physical fitness

(C) Nationality

(D) Literacy

(4) There are _____ types of health care reimbursement.

(A) 2

(B) 3

(C) 4

(D) 5

(5) What models are used for case management?

(A) Double case model

(B) ProACT model

(C) REACT model

(D) All of the above

(6) A patient who cannot speak or understand English fluently comes into the hospital. As a nurse, what is your next course of action?

(A) Find out what language the patient speaks and get an interpreter.

(B) Refer the patient based on language difference.

(C) Try to use signs to communicate.

(D) None of the above.

(7) Before performing a hysterectomy, a patient was properly counseled by a nurse on the implications, benefits, risks, side effects and alternatives. Then the client signed a document stating that she fully understood everything explained to her. What was displayed here?

(A) Consent

(B) Implied consent

(C) Informed consent

(D) All of the above

(8) A nurse that is not present during ward rounds cannot be said to be a good advocate for patients. This is because _____.

(A) Important decisions are made during the rounds

(B) The rounds show the nurse's commitment to getting promotions.

(C) Rounds are meant to give a chance for exercise and the nurse avoided extra exercise.

(D) The medical doctors will not be happy with the nurse for not being present during the rounds.


(9) What are some common referral needs?

(A) Social workers

(B) Self-help

(C) Shelters and housing

(D) All of the above

(10) What framework used in prioritization places physiological needs as a top priority?

(A) Resuscitation

(B) Maslow's Hierarchy of Needs

(C) Agency policies

(D) All of the above


(11) What areas benefit the most from performance improvement?

(A) Highest-risk areas

(B) Lowest-risk areas

(C) Lowest monetary areas

(D) None of the above


(12) What type of variance occurs when a part of the process is vulnerable to human error or is faulty?

(A) Random variance

(B) Specific variance

(C) Standard deviation

(D) All of the above

(13) What is currently the most popular performance improvement activity?

(A) PDCA cycle

(B) Six Sigma method

(C) Method de jour

(D) None of the above


(14) Which of the following are non-licensed?

(A) LPNs

(B) RNs

(C) Nursing assistants

(D) None of the above


(15) What specialty is primarily involved with a patient's functional abilities?

(A) Neurosurgeon

(B) Gynecology

(C) Physical therapists

(D) Occupational therapists

(16) Two of your nursing staff were involved in a conflict over working hours. The options to resolve this conflict are not completely satisfactory to both parties. According to Lewin, what type of conflict is this?

(A) Avoidance-Avoidance

(B) Avoidance-Acceptance

(C) Approach-Avoidance

(D) Double Approach-Avoidance


(17) Some of the most common causes of conflict in the health care setting include:

(A) Disrespect

(B) Overworking

(C) Ill health

(D) All of the above

(18) Multiple injured patients are brought to the emergency room. A patient sustained a fracture, major lacerations and bruises from an auto crash. What is your next line of action?

I – Inform doctors on call

II – Get materials ready for suturing

III – Administer ATS

IV – Refer the patient

(A) I, II, III

(B) I, II, IV

(C) I, III, II

(D) IV

(19) What should guide the delivery of health care?

(A) Pathophysiology

(B) Physiology

(C) Presentation

(D) All of the above

(20) A woman refuses immunization of her child for spiritual reasons. What should you do as a nurse?

(A) Counsel and educate her

(B) Document refusal

(C) A and B

(D) Immunize the child anyway.


(21) Fundamental responsibilities of a nurse include _____.

(A) Alleviating suffering

(B) Promoting health

(C) Preventing illness

(D) All of the above

(22) What is the right way to input information for clients?

(A) 09/10/20 1145 hrs. IV acetaminophen 900 mg stat given. Pain has subsided.

(B) 09/10/20 1145 hrs. IV acetaminophen 300 mg total dose given. Pain reported 2/10.

(C) 09/10/20 1145 hrs. IV acetaminophen given. The patient is feeling better.

(D) 09/10/20 1145 hrs. IV acetaminophen 300 mg STAT given. Patient reports pain as 2/10.

(23) You receive a call from one of your friends about her brother's wife, who has been admitted for two days. She wants to know what the diagnosis is. What should be your response?

(A) "Stop asking me these questions; it is against the law!"

(B) "I am sorry. I cannot give out such information about my clients."

(C) "What do you know about HIPAA?"

(D) Cut the call.

(24) A patient who only speaks Spanish comes to the emergency room. You are the nurse on duty and speak Spanish but are not fluent. What should you do?

(A) Speak English and use signs to ask the patient to leave.

(B) Speak Spanish and reassure the patient while you get an interpreter with a better command of the language

(C) Interpret as much as you can and hope the client understands.

(D) Refer the patient.

(25) A woman presents at the hospital with bruises and a black eye. You suspect physical abuse by her partner. She confides in you that it is true but asks you not to report it. What do you do?

(A) Follow her wishes.

(B) Document and report it.

(C) Scold the patient.

(D) Call her partner up to talk.

(26) Which of the following orders is most likely incorrect?

(A) IV acetaminophen 600 mg STAT for postoperative pain

(B) IV morphine 150 mg STAT for postoperative pain

(C) IV pentazocine 30 mg STAT for postoperative pain

(D) B and C


(27) A patient who has just suffered a stroke is brought into the emergency room. An urgent CT reveals a hemorrhagic stroke. What should be done next?

(A) Start medications.

(B) Look for relatives to sign the informed consent.

(C) Prepare for craniotomy.

(D) Admit the patient for bed rest.


(28) A 35-year-old woman presents with galactorrhea and has been experiencing a delay in conception. What targeted assessment would she benefit from?

(A) Complete blood count

(B) Nutritional assessment

(C) Hormonal profile

(D) All of the above

(29) Which of the following is false about high-risk behaviors?

(A) They are activities that increase the likelihood of harm.

(B) They are all modifiable.

(C) All risks are modifiable.

(D) None of the above.

(30) Which is not a major determinant of health risks?

(A) Age

(B) Socioeconomic status

(C) Hobbies

(D) None of the above

(31) What type of readiness to learn is most needed by a patient with a motor impairment who must start cleaning a wound appropriately?

(A) Experiential readiness

(B) Knowledge readiness

(C) Physical readiness

(D) All of the above

(32) What are some of the ways nurses can intervene in community health education?

(A) Oral presentations

(B) Policy approval

(C) Multidisciplinary cooperation

(D) A and C

(33) What is false about the New Ballard scale?

(A) It assesses physical and neuromuscular maturity.

(B) It is graded from 0 to 5.

(C) A scarf sign is a parameter.

(D) Heel-to-ear movement is a parameter.

(34) At what stage do disabilities affecting development become more obvious?

(A) Erikson's initiative vs. guilt stage

(B) Erikson's industry vs. inferiority stage

(C) Adolescence

(D) Toddler

(35) Which age group begins forming closer and stronger relationships with others?

(A) Young adults

(B) Middle age

(C) Elderly

(D) All of the above

(36) What are some of the musculoskeletal changes observed among the elderly?

(A) Increased muscle mass

(B) Increased intervertebral disc spaces

(C) Reduced muscle tone and strength

(D) B and C

(37) What is the EDD of a woman with LMP on March 20, 2023?

(A) November 25, 2023

(B) December 20, 2023

(C) December 25, 2023

(D) January 20, 2023

(38) What parameters are used to monitor a newborn's growth and development?

(A) OFC

(B) Length

(C) Feeding

(D) All of the above


(39) How often should the umbilical cord be cleaned after birth?

(A) Every hour

(B) Once every two days

(C) Weekly

(D) Several times a day


(40) As a nurse, how can you ensure a woman can breastfeed her baby correctly?

(A) Educate her.

(B) Breastfeed for her.

(C) Demonstrate it and let her watch you, then let her do it herself.

(D) Make sure she talks about breastfeeding a lot.

(41) Which of the following best describes the client care environment?

(A) The physical and social setting in which nursing care is provided

(B) The home environment of the client and the environment of the health care facility

(C) The environment of the health care facility alone

(D) The total of all the environments a client is exposed to

(42) To ensure a safe client care environment, the nurse should do all of the following except _____.

(A) Ensure the environment is safe from threats and potential hazards.

(B) Assess the quality of the client's home environment.

(C) Regulate the environment to minimize falls and injuries.

(D) Assess for and eliminate factors that can trigger self-harm in clients.

(43) What is the best method for signaling staff members about an unconscious patient's health state and safety in a private room?

(A) Bedside monitors

(B) Call bell

(C) An intercom system

(D) Communication boards

(44) Which of the following is not true about patient positioning methods?

(A) Clients should be supported and made comfortable in the Sim's position using pillows.

(B) The Sim's position is halfway between the prone position and the lateral position.

(C) The Sim's position is not the same as the semi-prone position.

(D) The Sim's position is not the same as the prone position.

(45) What is the recommended minimum number of identifiers assigned to each client?

(A) 1

(B) 2

(C) 3

(D) 4

(46) Which of the following can be classified as an internal disaster?

(A) A bomb blast that has occurred within the community

(B) A fire outbreak at a client's home

(C) A loaded truck that brings victims of a massive hurricane from a community nearby

(D) None of the above

(47) The principles of triage require that _____.

(A) The most critical situations be attended to first

(B) 10% of clients be discharged immediately if an emergency occurs

(C) The fittest clients are recruited to assist in attending to critical situations

(D) All of the above

(48) What is the right application of ergonomic principles in the health care environment?

(A) Using a specially designed wheelchair for transporting a client with a lumbar spine injury

(B) Helping clients decide the right assistive device to use for their unique needs

(C) Using tailored equipment for providing physiotherapy to individual clients

(D) All of the above


(49) Keeping your feet apart when lifting an object will help to _____.

(A) Channel all your strength into lifting the weight properly.

(B) Provide a secure base for better balance.

(C) Ensure your feet are not in the way of the other persons who are lifting the weight with you.

(D) All of the above.

(50) Which client would be more prone to repetitive stress injury?

(A) A client currently undergoing physiotherapy

(B) A client that mostly maintains the same position due to immobility or weakness in certain muscle groups

(C) A client that has been placed on bed rest for three days

(D) A client who exercises every day

(51) Why is it important for nurses to consider client pathophysiology when proffering home safety solutions?

(A) To ensure clients have the most minimal exposure to radiation

(B) To minimize exposure time

(C) To provide clients with the right procedures for handling biohazardous materials

(D) To ensure clients have an appropriate home environment for quick response and adjustment to new health challenges

(52) Which of the following are biohazardous materials?

(A) Sharp tools

(B) Used hospital beddings

(C) Cleaning agents

(D) Plastic wrappers

(53) What information should be included in formal reports for incidents and other irregular occurrences?

(A) The names of health care workers who were contacted to attend the event

(B) The date, time and place where the event occurred

(C) None of the above

(D) All of the above

(54) What are the different types of variances that should be recorded as irregular or out-of-place occurrences?

(A) Practitioner, system and institutional

(B) Patient, system and institutional

(C) Practitioner, system and patient

(D) None of the above

(55) What are transmission-based precautions?

(A) Measures taken to prevent the transfer of disease-causing organisms from one person or object to another

(B) Infection-control measures for preventing infection spread among clients, whether or not they've been diagnosed with any infection

(C) Preventive and infection-control measures utilized to combat and inhibit the spread of specific infections

(D) Specialized equipment used to protect specific body areas from injury and exposure to infectious agents


(56) The education of clients and staff members on infection prevention and control measures includes _____.

(A) Evaluating the impact and effectiveness of such educational sessions

(B) Assessing the educational needs of these people groups

(C) Planning educational activities to meet the unique educational needs of people

(D) All of the above

(57) Which of the following should not be done for immunocompromised clients to prevent them from contracting infection after exposure?

(A) Isolate them from other people until they have attained some level of recovery and immunity.

(B) Provide special care only when there is an infection outbreak.

(C) Utilize standard precautions when attending to them at all times.

(D) Prevent them from infections that might not pose a threat to non-compromised clients.


(58) What should nurses do if they need to cough or sneeze while working on a sterile field?

(A) Turn their backs to the sterile field and cough or sneeze.

(B) Cover their nose and mouth with their hands.

(C) Move away from the sterile field before coughing or sneezing.

(D) Cough or sneeze over the sterile field since they have a nose mask on.

(59) In which situations may restraints and safety devices be required?

(A) To prevent infection in patients

(B) To improve patient mobility

(C) To prevent safety threats such as falls

(D) To give patients a sense of autonomy


(60) Which of the following is not an appropriate type of restraint?

(A) Belts and jackets that prevent limb movement

(B) Holding down a patient

(C) Using medicine to keep the patient immobile

(D) Isolating the patient in one room without providing a means of exit


(61) Where would you check for the radial pulse?

(A) Lateral aspect of the arm

(B) Medial aspect of the arm

(C) Lateral aspect of the wrist

(D) Medial aspect of the wrist

(62) How much of the arm should the blood pressure cuff cover while checking for blood pressure?

(A) 1/2 of the upper arm

(B) 2/3 of the upper arm

(C) The entire arm

(D) 1/4 of the arm

(63) What equipment must match for blood glucose testing?

(A) Strip and lancet

(B) Meter and lancet

(C) Strip and meter

(D) All must match

(64) ECG leads are routinely placed on all the following parts of the body except the _____.

(A) Chest

(B) Hands

(C) Legs

(D) Head

(65) Why do we use standardized values?

(A) For competition among labs

(B) To compare with patient values

(C) To maintain the same values across laboratories

(D) All the above


(66) Why do we use a tourniquet in venipuncture?

(A) To arrest blood flow

(B) To engorge the veins

(C) To make the veins visible

(D) All of the above


(67) Urine can be routinely collected to investigate all of the following except
_____.

(A) Sexually transmitted infections

(B) Renal diseases

(C) Urinary tract infections

(D) Respiratory tract infections

(68) What is the role of a nurse to patients at risk?

(A) Identify them.

(B) Educate them.

(C) Refer them.

(D) A and B.

(69) A patient presents with skin cancer. What question should you not ask to rule out causes and major risk factors?

(A) Occupation

(B) Choice of diet

(C) Family history of skin cancer

(D) Personal history of skin cancer

(70) What are the initial signs to look out for when a patient might be hemorrhaging?

(A) Hypotension

(B) Hypertension

(C) Fever

(D) Pain

(71) What position is used in passing the NG tube in a conscious patient?

(A) Trendelenburg's position

(B) Left lateral decubitus position

(C) High Fowler's position

(D) Right lateral decubitus position

(72) At what angle should the needle be placed into the vein in IV cannulations?

(A) 20–40 degrees

(B) 10–20 degrees

(C) 45–90 degrees

(D) 15–30 degrees

(73) Which of the following must always be done before emptying the urine bag?

(A) Remove the catheter.

(B) Close the outlet.

(C) Note the volume of the urine.

(D) Pull the catheter to see if it's in place.

(74) Power in muscles is graded from _____.

(A) 1–5

(B) 2–10

(C) 0–5

(D) -1–6

(75) How many cranial nerves are present in the human body?

(A) 11

(B) 10

(C) 12

(D) 20

(76) Which of the following is false about therapeutic procedures?

(A) They're always medical.

(B) They can be surgical.

(C) They can be performed to remove foreign objects.

(D) They can be performed to repair wounds.

(77) What is the major role of the nurse in a surgical procedure?

(A) To help educate the client

(B) To help in moving the client

(C) To convince the patient

(D) All of the above

(78) Some diseases that are commonly transmitted by needle pricks include
_____.

(A) Hepatitis B

(B) Hepatitis A

(C) Leukemia

(D) All of the above

(79) What are coping mechanisms?

(A) Thoughts, behaviors, emotions

(B) Physiological adaptations of the heart

(C) Family patterns

(D) All of the above

(80) The most effective way to monitor bilirubin levels is _____.

(A) Checking for skin color

(B) Checking stool color

(C) Checking eye color

(D) Checking blood levels in the lab

(81) What are the types of needle biopsy?

(A) Fine needle aspiration and core needle biopsy

(B) Liver and lung biopsy

(C) Endoscopic biopsy and vacuum biopsy

(D) All of the above

(82) One basic technique to prevent infection in patients on a ventilator is _____.

(A) Antibiotics

(B) Blood culture

(C) Handwashing

(D) All of the above

(83) Which of the following statements is false?

(A) The tip of the suction catheter should be lubricated before advancing.

(B) Suctioning cannot be done more than once.

(C) Oxygen is given before suctioning.

(D) Only the nose can be suctioned.


(84) All of the following are examples of open wounds except _____.

(A) Abrasions

(B) Punctures

(C) Gunshot wounds

(D) Hematomas


(85) Patients who were under general anesthesia might feel exhausted and weak after they regain consciousness. What should the nurse do?

(A) Monitor vitals.

(B) Reassure the patients.

(C) Call the doctor for help.

(D) A and B.

(86) Postural drainage is most beneficial in all of the following conditions except
_____.

(A) COPD

(B) Bronchiectasis

(C) Lung abscess

(D) Acute rhinitis


(87) What are two types of dialysis?

(A) Hemodialysis and serodialysis

(B) Hemodialysis and perineal dialysis

(C) Hemodialysis and peritoneal dialysis

(D) Hemodialysis and renal transplant


(88) What organ function does dialysis replace?

(A) The kidneys' ultrafiltration function

(B) The liver's detoxification function

(C) The kidneys' hemopoietic function

(D) The kidneys' blood pressure regulation

(89) What stage of renal failure is an indication for dialysis?

(A) Stage II

(B) Stage III

(C) Stage IV

(D) Stage V


(90) Which is the most abundant extracellular cation?

(A) Cl

(B) Na

(C) K

(D) Mg


(91) Which of the following is not involved in either muscular or cardiac contractions?

(A) Na

(B) K

(C) Ca

(D) None of the above

(92) A patient is observed to be dyspneic, with edema of the lower and upper limbs. He is on an infusion of normal saline. His blood pressure is elevated. What is the first line of action?

(A) Stop the fluid infusion.

(B) Commence Lasix.

(C) Adjust the position.

(D) Reduce the fluid infusion.

(93) What is the first line of treatment in hypovolemia?

(A) Suturing

(B) Resuscitation

(C) Fluid restriction

(D) None of the above

(94) Arterial lines cannot be placed in the _____.

(A) Femoral artery

(B) Brachial artery

(C) Radial artery

(D) Common interosseous artery

(95) What are some of the complications of a pacemaker?

(A) Pneumothorax

(B) Hemothorax

(C) Cardiac tamponade

(D) All of the above

(96) Which of the following is easily done with the knowledge of the heart's electrical impulse?

(A) Interpretation of blood sugar values

(B) Interpretation of ECG

(C) Interpretation of EEG

(D) All of the above

(97) Patients should be given a good education on any disease condition they have. This information should include disease _____.

(A) Pathophysiology

(B) Etiology

(C) Signs and symptoms

(D) All of the above

(98) Why must nurses explain the signs and symptoms of a disease to clients?

(A) For prompt self-medication

(B) For prompt presentation at the hospital as necessary

(C) To educate others with a similar condition

(D) B and C


(99) Features of hypernatremia do not include _____.

(A) Thirst

(B) Agitation

(C) Restlessness and confusion

(D) Arrhythmias


(100) You are the nurse on duty in a ward. Which of the following patients is at the most risk of developing bed sores?

(A) An elderly patient with hypertension

(B) An elderly patient with a history of cigarette smoking

(C) An elderly patient with heart failure

(D) An elderly patient with well-treated diabetes mellitus

(101) A patient is identified as having possible mobility issues during admission. As the admitting nurse, what are the appropriate initial steps you should take in evaluating the patient?

(A) Giving the patient instructions to evaluate movement

(B) Observation of the patient for signs of immobility

(C) Reading through the patient's history and examination findings

(D) Running a quick physical examination of mobility


(102) A patient on chronic opioid medication for cancer is noticed to be dependent on the opioid. What is the best next line of action?

(A) Reprimand the patient.

(B) Withdraw the opioid medication.

(C) Assess the patient with the CAGE questionnaire.

(D) Document the issue and inform relatives.

(103) Your patient is to be commenced on nonpharmacological treatment for severe pain. Which of the following is not a modality of nonpharmacological treatment in the management of pain?

(A) Art

(B) Massage

(C) Companionship

(D) Dietary modification

(104) A patient who is being treated for septicemia is noticed to have an adverse drug reaction to the medications he is on. The patient is on the following medications: aspirin, gentamicin and hydrochlorothiazide. Which of the following evaluations is most appropriate for recognizing the adverse drug reaction?

(A) Speech assessment

(B) Hearing assessment

(C) Visual assessment

(D) Mobility assessment

(105) A patient is admitted to the nephrology ward and is being managed for a renal condition. Which of the following is not a primary renal/urinary tract complaint?

(A) Polyuria

(B) Frequency

(C) Urgency

(D) Polydipsia


(106) An 80-year-old presents to the ER with acute urinary retention secondary to bladder outlet obstruction due to benign enlargement of the prostate. The urinary retention is to be relieved by passing a urinary catheter. Which of the following is not ideal during the procedure?

(A) Passage of lidocaine gel into the urethra before catheterization

(B) Inflation of the self-retaining catheter after passage

(C) Adequate draping of phallus before catheterization

(D) Use of a smaller-sized urinary catheter to prevent pain and discomfort

(107) A patient has a pelvic fracture following a traffic accident. Which of the following devices is the most appropriate for mobilization?

(A) Overhead trapeze bar

(B) Wheelchair

(C) Zimmer's walking frame

(D) Axillary crutches

(108) A patient with advanced gastric cancer had gastric bypass surgery and is experiencing dumping syndrome. Which counsel is contraindicated in this patient?

(A) Small frequent meals

(B) Intake of high glucose content meal

(C) Intake of food rich in fiber

(D) Moderation of fluid intake with meals

(109) A preterm neonate admitted to the neonatal intensive unit is noticed to be excessively calm and shows reduced activity. Which of the following is not the most likely cause of this?

(A) Hypoglycemia

(B) Hypothermia

(C) Hypocalcemia

(D) Hypoxia


(110) A 65-year-old man was admitted for hip surgery following a hip fracture. Which of the following is not an anticipated respiratory complication of prolonged immobilization?

(A) Pulmonary fibrosis

(B) Atelectasis

(C) Hypostatic pneumonia

(D) Respiratory tract infections

(111) A seven-year-old boy is being managed for severe Guillain-Barré syndrome. Which system is not anticipated to be affected by the prolonged immobilizations associated with this condition?

(A) Integumentary

(B) Neurological

(C) Musculoskeletal

(D) Gastrointestinal

(112) Meg has been acting aggressively over her last two clinic visits. She flares up whenever the nurse tells her she cannot get a higher dose of antidepressants than she is taking. She keeps saying the medicine is not working; she says she needs more to stay calm and gets angry when she does not take her drugs. What is the likely diagnosis?

(A) Physical dependence

(B) Substance abuse

(C) Drug-seeking behavior

(D) All of the above

(113) What is not a major risk factor for substance abuse?

(A) Low pain threshold

(B) High pain threshold

(C) Mental disorder

(D) High risk-taking tendencies

(114) Which of the following factors are not considered in evaluating a substance abuse client's response to a treatment plan?

(A) Achieving sobriety

(B) Client participation in therapy

(C) Prevention of falls

(D) Response to medications

(115) A young woman lost her child a month ago and is very angry at her husband. She blames him for not taking her baby to the hospital in time while she was away to see a friend. She also blames her friend for not turning down her offer to visit since she was still nursing her baby. What coping mechanism is being displayed here?

(A) Regression

(B) Compensation

(C) Displacement

(D) Intellectualization

(116) Liz wrote a suicide note, which her husband found. He called her friend, who persuaded her to visit the hospital. What is your first line of action?

(A) Use restraints on Liz.

(B) Place her on observation.

(C) Begin therapy right away.

(D) Refer Liz to a psychotherapist.

(117) While attending to your patient, you wave at a colleague and observe that your patient is very uncomfortable with your gesture. It happens twice when you wave. What do you do?

(A) Apologize for making her uncomfortable and ask what the gesture means to her

(B) Continue as if nothing happened

(C) Find out what the gesture means to her and apologize if need be

(D) Stop waving while attending to the patient

(118) What are some of the end-of-life concerns that patients have?

(A) Fear of the unknown

(B) Fear of choices made

(C) What will become of the family when they are gone

(D) All of the above

(119) A type of family structure where the leader makes all the decisions with little or no room for deliberation is _____.

(A) Democratic

(B) Laissez-faire

(C) Authoritarian

(D) None of the above


(120) Which of the following is not related to grief and loss?

(A) Worden's four tasks

(B) Engel's stages

(C) Sander's phases

(D) Anna's phases


(121) Lack of insight is an indication of _____.

(A) Self-efficacy

(B) Internal locus of control

(C) Possible non-adherence to the treatment plan

(D) Adherence to the treatment plan

(122) What is one important trait a nurse must exhibit while caring for patients with perception alterations?

(A) Acuity

(B) Patience

(C) Sound judgment

(D) Nonjudgmental disposition

(123) Examples of nonverbal cues that a nurse must learn to recognize to manage stress effectively include _____.

(A) Pupil dilation

(B) Increased respiratory rate

(C) Sluggish movement

(D) All of the above

(124) Methods of clarification include _____.

(A) Restating, paraphrasing, reflecting

(B) Challenging, probing, disagreeing

(C) Focusing, paraphrasing, restating

(D) Changing subject, judgment, stereotyping

(125) Concerning the different compatibilities of drugs, which of the following is false?

(A) Not all drugs have drug-drug interactions.

(B) Compatible drugs can be supplied in the same syringe without risk.

(C) All of the above.

(D) None of the above.

(126) You are to administer an oil- and water-based medication intramuscularly. What is the best way to approach this?

(A) Administer both separately.

(B) Mix both in the same syringe.

(C) Give one intramuscularly and the other subcutaneously.

(D) None of the above.

(127) Adverse drug reactions can be _____.

(A) Dose-related

(B) Time-related

(C) All of the above

(D) None of the above

(128) All of the following are blood transfusion reactions except _____.

(A) Fever

(B) Chills and rigor

(C) Tachycardia

(D) Tachyphonia


(129) What hematological test is most important before a patient is transfused with fresh whole blood?

(A) Full blood count and differential

(B) Blood type and antigen screen

(C) Grouping and crossmatching

(D) Blood culture

(130) While monitoring a patient getting fresh whole blood, he suddenly complains of respiratory distress. Upon checking his vital signs, you notice both his heart rate and blood pressure are elevated. Your auscultatory findings are bibasal crackles. What issue is the client most likely dealing with?

 (A) Transfusion reaction

(B) Pulmonary embolism

(C) Myocardial ischemia

(D) Circulatory overload

(131) Which of the following veins are not useful for central venous access?

(A) Subclavian

(B) Jugular

(C) Superior vena cava

(D) Inferior vena cava

(132) All of the following are complications of central venous access except
_____.

(A) Hemothorax

(B) Venous ulcers

(C) Pneumothorax

(D) Embolism

(133) The nurse assesses the insertion site on a central line. Which finding needs to be further investigated?

(A) Biopatch and transparent dressing

(B) A small amount of dried blood

(C) Both A & B

(D) Erythema and tenderness

(134) _____ need(s) the highest level of accuracy in dosing and administration.

(A) Drug therapy in pediatrics

(B) Intravenous fluids

(C) Food

(D) Vitamins

(135) What is the equivalent volume of 500 ml in pints?

(A) 0.5 pints

(B) 1 pint

(C) 2 pints

(D) 4 pints

(136) What is the most common and convenient route of drug administration?

(A) Buccal route

(B) Intravenous route

(C) Transdermal route

(D) Oral route

(137) Which of the following should the nurse not tell a patient about verifying the medication's label?

(A) Name of the medication

(B) Dose of the medication

(C) Expiry date of the medication

(D) None of the above

(138) A patient is brought to the emergency department with third-degree burns. What is the appropriate mode of nutrition for this patient?

(A) Oral feeding

(B) Tube feeding

(C) Hyperalimentation

(D) Bottle feeding

(139) What are the main reasons for using total parenteral nutrition?

(A) Complete bowel rest, negative nitrogen balance, serious medical illness or disease

(B) Convenience

(C) Athletic performance improvement

(D) Routine health maintenance

(140) What is the purpose of a hyperalimentation catheter?

(A) To deliver total parenteral nutrition

(B) To improve athletic performance

(C) To replace regular meals for convenience

(D) To cure diseases

(141) What are opioids used for in pain management?

(A) Mild pain

(B) Moderate to severe pain

(C) Chronic pain

(D) Emotional pain

(142) What are some common side effects of opioid medications?

(A) Drowsiness, constipation and nausea

(B) Increased energy and alertness

(C) Increased appetite and weight gain

(D) Increased blood pressure and heart rate

(143) What is the goal of pain management?

(A) To eliminate all pain

(B) To ignore pain

(C) To minimize pain to a tolerable level

(D) To maximize pain for emotional distress

(144) Which of the following is not a potential risk of opioid medications?

(A) Addiction

(B) Constipation

(C) Lowered blood pressure

(D) Respiratory depression

(145) A patient is rushed to the emergency department. The patient is groaning in pain as he has a fractured arm. Which of the following pain management techniques is most appropriate for this patient?

(A) Use of non-opioids

(B) Use of opioids

(C) Cold therapy

(D) Psychotherapy

(146) What are some common complications of intravenous infusion therapy?

(A) Hemorrhage and emboli

(B) Infections and phlebitis

(C) Allergic reactions and anaphylaxis

(D) Nausea and vomiting

(147) What is the significance of selecting an appropriate vein for patients requiring a blood transfusion via intravenous catheter?

(A) To minimize the risk of hematoma

(B) To prevent fluid overload

(C) To avoid allergic reactions

(D) To ensure a successful blood transfusion

(148) Why is critical thinking crucial for RNs regarding medications?

(A) Patients can be sensitive to medications.

(B) Medication administration can be complex.

(C) Medication side effects can be severe.

(D) All of the above.

(149) What are the side effects of medications?

(A) Desired therapeutic impacts

(B) Allergic reactions

(C) Consequences of a drug that are not expected

(D) Severe adverse effects

(150) Patients respond differently to medications for all of the following reasons except _____.

(A) Age

(B) Health status

(C) Eye color

(D) Individual variability in drug metabolism

# Test 3: Answers and Explanations

(1) (B) Self-Determination Act.

The Self-Determination Act was passed by Congress in 1990. It gives patients the right to either accept or reject care on admission to any health care facility. This act also gives patients the right to ask for advance directives.

(2) (B) The nurse delegating retains no responsibility for the outcome of the delegated task.

This is not true. Delegation means a task is given to another person to perform. In the nursing profession, delegation means a nurse transfers a responsibility or task to another nursing staff member but retains responsibility for the outcome of the task.

(3) (A) Skills and knowledge.

Skills and knowledge qualify a person for a job. An RN must assign jobs on this basis. Tasks must be given to staff based on the skills that they possess. There must be no sentiment about this because if a member of staff is assigned a job without possessing the skills to perform it, they may deliver poor quality care to the client and could make themselves and the delegating nurse liable for legal action.

(4) (A) 2.

There are two types of health care reimbursement: prospective and retrospective.

(5) (B) ProACT model.

The Robert Wood Johnson University Hospital created this model of case management. Other models are the collaborative practice model, the case manager model and the triad model of case management.

(6) (A) Find out what language the patient speaks and get an interpreter.

Every client has the right to accurate and easy-to-understand information about the plan for their health. Clients must know what is happening at every point in their care. If there is a communication barrier, such as a language difference, an interpreter should be provided to ensure clients understand clearly what is being done.

(7) (C) Informed consent.

Informed consent means that patients must give full consent to whatever procedures or treatment plans are recommended, with full knowledge of the proposed treatment, including the benefits, risks, side effects, recovery, alternatives, etc.

(8) (A) Important decisions are made during the rounds.

Advocacy cannot happen if the nurse is absent. This is more important when critical decisions are being made, for instance, during rounds. Patients spend more time with nurses and, as such, are more comfortable discussing their concerns with them. So, the RNs can discuss these concerns with doctors or other health care workers involved in patient management. However, this can only happen when they are present.

(9) (D) All of the above.

A nurse must be able to recognize the appropriate resources for common referral needs. Examples are anger management programs, social workers, self-help groups in the community for those who battle addiction or other mental health conditions, shelters and housing for clients who might be abuse victims, and elderly day care for older patients.

(10) (B) Maslow's hierarchy of needs.

Maslow's hierarchy of needs shows that the first thing to attend to is the patient's physiological needs, then safety, security, self-esteem and self-actualization.

(11) (A) Highest risk areas.

The best areas for quality improvement are those with the highest risk, monetary and human resource costs, volume and most vulnerable to problems. Performance improvement aims at enhancing and improving the quality and outcomes of care, increasing the efficiency of patient care while reducing costs, risks and liabilities.

(12) (B) Specific variance.

A specific variance occurs whenever the faulty process is carried out. It is predictable and usually occurs when a specific part of the process is faulty or vulnerable to human error.

(13) (C) Method de jour.

Performance improvement activities can be done through many methods, some of which include the PDCA cycle, which involves Planning, Doing, Checking and Acting; the Six Sigma method, which involves problem definition measuring, analysis of data, improvements to make and control; and the method de jour.

(14) (C) Nursing assistants.

LPNs are licensed health care professionals. They provide a wide variety of nursing care services in many different health care settings. RNs are licensed health care personnel who are trained to deliver nursing care in several health care settings. Nursing assistants/patient care technicians are non-licensed assistants who help nurses to provide direct and indirect care.

(15) (C) Physical therapists.

Physical therapists are licensed health care personnel that provide medical interventions concerned with a patient's functional abilities. They consider factors like strength, gait and mobility and use tools like walkers and exercise routines to achieve their outcomes.

(16) (C) Approach-Avoidance.

Here, the choices that can resolve the conflict are not completely satisfactory to both parties, but neither are they completely unsatisfactory.

(17) (D) All of the above.

Some of the most common causes of conflict in health care settings are disrespect, overworking, unfair distribution of roles or duties, ill health, patient loss, negligence, limited resources, poor remuneration, poor communication skills and different personality types.

(18) (C) I, III, II.

Doctors on call should be informed. Anti-tetanus serum/tetanus toxoid should be given, and materials for suturing should be prepared. The patient also requires an X-ray.

(19) (A) Pathophysiology.

The pathophysiology of the disease should guide the delivery of care. The presentation is important but does not always determine how care is administered. Some presentations might be dramatic but not urgent. Some patients also exaggerate their symptoms. Hence, understanding disease conditions should guide how care is delivered, not subjective displays or responses.

(20) (C) A and B.

Scenarios like this should be documented, including the counseling and the refusal, and reported to appropriate authorities for follow-up. A nurse should not forcefully immunize a child against the wishes of the parents and caregiver. The parent is the major consent giver for minors.

(21) (D) All of the above.

The fundamental responsibility of the nurse is to prevent illness, promote health, restore health and alleviate suffering.

(22) (D) 09/10/20 1145 hrs. IV acetaminophen 300 mg STAT given. Patient reports pain as 2/10.

The right way to input information for clients is the date, time, drug and correct route of administration, dose, frequency and assessment of the patient.

(23) (B) "I am sorry. I cannot give out such information about my clients."

Let your friend know that you cannot give out such information. It is against HIPAA to give out information to a person whose input is not necessary to the care of the patient, either directly or indirectly. Suggest your friend call and ask her brother or his wife.

(24) (B) Speak Spanish and reassure the patient while you get an interpreter with a better command of the language.

You should allow the patient to calm down by speaking whatever Spanish is possible. Then you can go get an interpreter with a better command of the language. If you go ahead and try and interpret, there might be a misunderstanding or a loss of the message to be passed across.

(25) (B) Document and report it.

Abuse of clients, gunshot wounds, road traffic accidents, burns, harmful diseases or cases of food poisoning should be reported. VOs can only be used during emergencies. Since this is not an emergency, the physician can request another physician who is around to document the order so it can be given.

(26) (B) IV morphine 150 mg STAT for postoperative pain.

Most likely this is an incorrect dosage. IV morphine is usually given between 4 mg to 10 mg over three or four times daily or PRN. The dose of 150 mg STAT is not correct.

(27) (C) Prepare for craniotomy.

Informed consent is not needed when a delay would cause harm or death to the patient. In this case, looking around for the patient's relatives can result in a waste of precious time. This patient needs to receive care as soon as possible. The law allows this kind of scenario without informed consent.

(28) (C) Hormonal profile.

A hormonal profile test is a blood test that is used to detect hormonal imbalances and fertility issues in women. It assesses the quantity of estrogen, progesterone, thyroid hormones, follicle-stimulating hormone and testosterone. For this case, a doctor might also include prolactin as one of the hormones to test for.

(29) (C) All risks are modifiable.

Biologically, some risks are evident based on race, age and gender and cannot be modified. For instance, the female gender has a higher chance of breast cancer than the male gender.

(30) (D) None of the above.

There are several health risks that individuals are exposed to daily. Some of these risks are based on the patients' age, socioeconomic status, hobbies, lifestyle choices, location and population. It is the nurse's responsibility to assess clients for possible health risks that they are exposed to knowingly or unknowingly.

(31) (C) Physical readiness.

Physical readiness involves the measures of ability, the complexity of the task, the effect of the environment, the health status of the individual and gender. The measures of physical ability determine whether a patient is ready to learn or not. A patient with a motor impairment might find it difficult to perform some fine movements and might not be ready to learn things such as cleaning a surgical wound appropriately.

(32) (D) A and C.

From time to time, nurses have to provide education to help achieve these objectives of developing health characteristics. When these needs are identified, the nurse can devise a plan to intervene as needed. It might involve educating community members via oral presentations, counseling and guidance for individuals or even multidisciplinary cooperation to intervene. Policy approval is not the duty of a nurse.

(33) (B) It is graded from 0 to 5.

This scale is based on both physical maturity and the maturity of the neuromuscular system. It is graded from -1 to 5 and measures the following parameters: posture, square window, which refers to the movement of the wrist, arm recoil, scarf sign and heel-to-ear movement.

(34) (A) Erikson's initiative vs. guilt stage.

Erikson's initiative vs. guilt stage coincides with the preschooler age (three to five years). At this stage, children are refining motor skills. This is the stage at which disabilities affecting development are more obvious.

(35) (A) Young adults.

Young adults between 19 and 35 are at the intimacy vs. isolation stage, according to Erikson. Here, they begin to form closer, stronger relationships with other people. This stage is also characterized by seeking purpose in life and developing healthy coping mechanisms to deal with the demands of work, relationships and other commitments.

(36) (D) B and C.

Musculoskeletal changes in the elderly include a decrease in muscle mass, muscle tone and strength, degenerating joints, bones and reductions in intervertebral disc spaces.

(37) (C) December 25, 2023.

The EDD is calculated as 40 weeks after the last menstrual period (LMP). It can be used in clinical settings to estimate the EDD. However, the most reliable method of estimating the EDD is the early ultrasound taken in the first trimester of pregnancy.

(38) (D) All of the above.

The OFC of the newborn should increase at an average rate of 2 cm per month for the first three months, then 1 cm per month for the next six months. The length should also increase at a rate of about 2.5 cm per month for the first six months and about 1.3 cm for the last six months of the first year. If a child is not feeding well, it should be checked as soon as possible.

(39) (D) Several times a day.

The umbilical cord stump usually falls off a newborn within one to two weeks after birth. Until it falls off, the area should be kept clean and dry, and it should be cleaned several times a day. This helps prevent infection. After each diaper change, the area around the cord should be cleaned with a cotton swab dipped in warm water, then dried thoroughly.

(40) (C) Demonstrate it and let her watch you, then let her do it herself.

This is false. The only way to ascertain for sure that a woman is breastfeeding her child right is to watch her do it, especially if this is her first child. This type of learning ensures that the mother uses the right technique that will not harm her or the baby over time.

(41) (A) The physical and social setting in which nursing care is provided.

The client care environment refers to the physical and social setting in which nursing care is provided. Assessing the client care environment involves taking into consideration factors such as safety, comfort, privacy and cultural sensitivity.

(42) (B) Assess the quality of the client's home environment.

The environment must be regulated to minimize falls and other injuries to ensure a safe client care environment. Materials and equipment used should be sterile or properly disinfected before reuse, and all allergens must be removed. The environment should also be checked for factors that can trigger self-harm or aggression in patients.

(43) (A) Bedside monitors.

Bedside monitors are the most effective for monitoring clients who are unconscious and unable to use other methods for signaling staff members.

(44) (C) The Sim's position is not the same as the semi-prone position.

This is false. The Sim's position is also known as the semi-prone position and is halfway between the prone and lateral positions.

(45) (B) 2.

Having at least two distinct identifiers for each client besides their room number is recommended.

(46) (D) None of the above.

Internal disasters are those that occur within the confines of medical facilities, such as fire hazards, workplace violence, radiation contamination, building collapse and other utility failures.

(47) (A) The most critical situations be attended to first.

During triage, the nurse should assess patients' situations from most critical to least critical. Critical situations should be attended to first, and in situations of equipment and bed space shortage, non-critical patients may be treated and discharged immediately.

(48) (D) All of the above.

Ergonomic principles can be applied when providing health care. These will help offer comfort to clients and help them maintain the right posture, balance, body alignment and body movement when they are using assistive devices and other facilities like beds and stretchers. Nurses should keep in mind ergonomic principles and body mechanics when providing care to clients and helping them use assistive devices.

(49) (B) Provide a secure base for better balance.

Keeping your feet apart helps provide a secure base for supporting yourself when lifting.

(50) (B) A client that mostly maintains the same position due to immobility or weakness in certain muscle groups.

Clients that maintain the same position over time have a high risk of repetitive stress injury due to the overuse of certain muscles or muscle groups.

(51) (D) To ensure clients have an appropriate home environment for quick response and adjustment to new health challenges.

Nurses must strongly consider client pathophysiology and the uniqueness of each client's situation when offering solutions to ensure clients have an appropriate home environment for quick response and adjustment to new health challenges.

(52) (B) Used hospital bedding.

Biohazardous material includes items that have been contaminated with biological waste that can become harmful to humans. Used hospital beddings, tubes containing bodily fluids and excretions and used needles are all examples of biohazardous waste.

(53) (D) All of the above.

Details that should be included in formal reports include the date, time and place where the event happened, brief background information on what triggered the event, the name of people affected by the event and the nature of the injuries sustained.

(54) (C) Practitioner, system and patient.

The events that should be reported include practitioner variance, system or institutional variance and patient variance.

(55) (C) Preventive and infection control measures utilized to combat and inhibit the spread of specific infections.

Transmission-based precautions are additional infection prevention measures used for patients with known or suspected infectious diseases, which are based on the disease's mode of transmission.

(56) (D) All of the above.

RNs directly and indirectly educate clients and staff members on infection prevention and control measures. They assess the educational needs of these groups and plan educational activities to meet those needs. They also evaluate the impact and effectiveness of such educational sessions on infection prevention and control.

(57) (B) Provide special care only when there is an infection outbreak.

Immunocompromised clients should be isolated from other people until they have attained some level of recovery and immunity, and stringent infection control measures should be practiced, including protecting them from infections that might not pose a threat to non-compromised clients.

(58) (C) Move away from the sterile field before coughing or sneezing.

Coughing or sneezing over the sterile field contaminates it, so the nurse should move away from the sterile field before coughing or sneezing. The nurse should never have the sterile field below the waist level. The nurse leans over or turns their back to the sterile field.

(59) (C) To prevent safety threats such as falls.

Restraints and safety devices may be required when mobility can increase the risk of falls, suicide attempts or causing harm to others.

(60) (D) Isolating the patient in one room without providing a means of exit.

Different kinds of restraints can be used depending on the situation. These include using belts, jackets and other devices to prevent limb movement, holding down a patient to restrict movement and using medicine to keep the patient immobile. However, isolating the patient in one room without providing a means of exit is not an appropriate type of restraint.

(61) (C) Lateral aspect of the wrist.

Knowledge of the anatomy of the body and the pathophysiology of diseases is critical in noticing and responding to abnormal vital signs. For instance, knowledge of anatomy helps a nurse read the radial pulse on the lateral side of the wrist. The radial pulse gives the pulse rate of the individual. The average in an adult is 70 bpm.

(62) (B) 2/3 of the upper arm.

While there are varying schools of thought, what is recommended in most textbooks and experience from practitioners is two-thirds of the upper arm's length. This upper arm length is defined as the distance between the axilla and the antecubital fossa. A wrong cuff size can affect the result of the blood pressure measurement.

(63) (C) Strip and meter.

The nurse should use the right strip and meter to do blood glucose testing.

(64) (D) Head.

ECG leads are placed on the upper limbs, chest and lower limbs.

(65) (B) To compare with patient values.

Standardized values are essential in laboratory investigations. They form a baseline with which we can compare patient values for the determination of quantities that are depressed, normal or elevated. They also help to monitor values and determine if the treatment plan is beneficial to the patient or not.

(66) (D) All of the above.

A tourniquet is used in venipuncture to briefly arrest blood flow back to the heart, making the veins engorged and more visible so that the cannula can be easily inserted. The tourniquet is also used to ensure the skin is taut around the region for the venipuncture.

(67) (D) Respiratory tract infections.

Urine is routinely collected for urinary tract infections, sexually transmitted infections and renal diseases. Urine is not routinely collected for investigations of respiratory tract infections.

(68) (D) A and B.

After identifying these patients, nurses are responsible for educating them on how to avoid complications of their diseases and avoid developing others they are at risk of. This education includes lifestyle choices and their impact, which can be immediate, temporary, longer or permanent.

(69) (B) Choice of diet.

Patients with a family history or relatives with skin cancer are also at risk. Patients whose occupation exposes them to ultraviolet radiation are also predisposed to skin cancers. Patients with a personal history of skin cancer are at risk. No significant study links diet as a major risk factor for skin cancer.

(70) (A) Hypotension.

Hypotension refers to the falling of blood pressure below normal values, usually less than 90/60 mmHg. Hypertension with a corresponding pulse might later happen when the body is trying to adapt. Patients might also experience confusion, weakness, blurring of vision or fainting.

(71) (C) High Fowler's position.

In this position, the patient is seated upright with the upper body positioned between 60 and 90 degrees. This position greatly reduces the risk of regurgitation and aspiration.

(72) (D) 15–30 degrees.

At 15–30 degrees, the cannula can be easily advanced into the vein. This angle also allows for easy visualization of the flashback of blood once the cannula gets into the vein.

(73) (C) Note the volume of the urine.

Removal of the catheter must be done using aseptic techniques. Most importantly, the catheter should be removed gently, disconnected from the urine bag and properly disposed of. The contents must be measured before the bag is emptied.

(74) (C) 0–5.

The nurse can assess the muscles and score them from 0–5. The muscles score zero if there's no visible contraction and score five (full power) if there's a full contraction against high resistance levels. A zero score can be due to either neurological or musculoskeletal anomalies.

(75) (C) 12.

The 12 cranial nerves include the olfactory nerve (CN I); the optic nerve (CN II); the oculomotor nerve (CN III); the trochlear nerve (CN IV); the trigeminal nerve (CN V); the abducens nerve (CN VI); the facial nerve (CN VII); the vestibulocochlear nerve (CN VIII); the glossopharyngeal nerve (CN IX); the vagus nerve (CN X); the spinal accessory nerve (CN XI) and the hypoglossal nerve (CN XII).

(76) (A) They're always medical.

Therapeutic procedures are not always medical. The modality of the therapeutic procedure employed depends on the condition. But surgical procedures are sometimes the only form of therapy that can address a condition, such as tumors.

(77) (A) To help educate the client.

Educating the client about the treatment procedure is a skill every nurse should know. A nurse should explain each procedure's benefits, risks and side effects. Every patient also has the right to forfeit or reject a treatment. Lastly, a nurse must get informed consent before starting a treatment.

(78) (A) Hepatitis B.

Hepatitis B is the only illness in this question transmitted by needle pricks. Hepatitis A is transmitted by the fecal-oral route. Leukemia is a disease of the white blood cells, which can be due to several etiologies, but not needle pricks. Other diseases that can be transmitted by needle pricks include HIV/AIDS and Hepatitis C.

(79) (A) Thoughts, behaviors, emotions.

Coping mechanisms are thoughts, behaviors and emotions that patients use to adapt to and cope with stress. Some of these mechanisms can be healthy, while others are maladaptive.

(80) (D) Checking blood levels in the lab.

All other ways are subjective and can be affected by lighting conditions, the nurse's experience and the baby's skin color. But the blood levels of bilirubin shown by lab tests can accurately tell if the bilirubin levels are elevated or not. In the clinical setting, other methods, such as the skin color and color of the eyes, can be used to detect hyperbilirubinemia, but they must be confirmed by a bilirubin test.

(81) (A) Fine needle aspiration and core needle biopsy.

Fine needle aspiration (FNA) is a minimally invasive diagnostic procedure that involves the insertion of a fine hollow needle into a mass or lump for the purpose of obtaining samples, which are then stained and observed. Core needle biopsy is also an invasive diagnostic procedure that uses a slightly larger needle to obtain more tissue from masses. It is generally preferred to the FNA.

(82) (C) Handwashing.

Bacteria and microbes can hide in the inner lining of ventilator tubes and cause infections in patients. Pneumonia is a common disease acquired by patients on ventilators. Basic aseptic techniques like handwashing can prevent the transfer of bacteria to patients.

(83) (B) Suctioning cannot be done more than once.

This is false. Suctioning is the mechanical aspiration of pulmonary secretions from the airways. Oxygen is administered before suctioning to maintain the airways during suctioning. A sterile glove is worn, and the tip of the suction catheter is lubricated. The catheter is slowly advanced into the patient's airways to remove secretions. This process can be repeated until the airways are clear.

(84) (D) Hematomas.

A hematoma refers to a collection of blood, mostly clotted in a closed cavity or space. Hematomas usually result from the rupture of an artery or vein within a tissue, an organ or a cavity. Hematomas can form a lump under the skin which can be felt, but they are not open wounds. Abrasions, punctures and gunshot wounds are all open wounds.

(85) (D) A and B.

The patient is monitored after surgery by the nurse. The vital signs are first examined. The pulse rate and blood pressure are measured. The respiratory system is also examined. Patients recovering from general anesthesia are at risk of dysphagia and laryngospasms. They might also feel some lightheadedness and drowsiness, which will eventually wear off. So patients should be reassured.

(86) (D) Acute rhinitis.

Postural drainage is very useful in patients with conditions that produce excessive secretions, such as COPD or bronchiectasis. Acute rhinitis does not produce copious secretions and is not an indication of postural drainage.

(87) (C) Hemodialysis and peritoneal dialysis.

Dialysis replaces the function of the kidney. There are two types of dialysis—hemodialysis and peritoneal dialysis. Hemodialysis is a form of dialysis via an AV fistula or a central vascular line. An AV is a connection between an artery and vein and is done three months before the dialysis to allow for maturity. Peritoneal dialysis is done by passing a catheter into the peritoneal space. This option is for patients who are at risk of complications from medications given on hemodialysis.

(88) (A) The kidneys' ultrafiltration function.

As a result of failure, the kidneys cannot filter waste products for excretion. Therefore, waste products accumulate in the body, which is dangerous to the patient. Dialysis helps to remove these waste products. It replaces the ultrafiltration function of the kidneys by clearing waste products from the body and balancing the pH of the blood.

(89) (D) Stage V.

There are five stages of renal failure or chronic kidney disease. Stage I presents with a normal GFR of 90 ml/min or higher. Stage II is mild CKD with GR of 60–89 ml/min. Stage III is moderate CKD with GFR of 30–59 ml/min. Stage 4 is Severe CKD with GFR of 15–29 ml/min. Stage 5 is the end stage CKD with GFR of < 15 ml/min. End-stage CKD is where dialysis or renal transplant is needed.

(90) (B) Na.

Sodium (Na) is the most abundant extracellular cation, and it is heavily involved in muscular contraction. Potassium (K) is the most abundant intracellular cation. Magnesium is a dominant intracellular ion that also regulates several signaling pathways and channels. It is also involved in preventing continuous muscular contractions. Chlorine is an anion.

(91) (D) None of the above.

Sodium and potassium are the major cations involved in muscular contraction, while calcium is involved in both cardiac and muscular contraction.

(92) (A) Stop the fluid infusion.

The patient is most likely suffering from fluid overload due to the infusion that is being received. Therefore, the first step is to stop the infusion. The next step would be to commence the patient on Lasix.

(93) (B) Resuscitation.

Fluid resuscitation is the first line of treatment in hypovolemia. Infusion of intravenous fluids like ringer's lactate can expand the blood volume.

(94) (D) Common interosseous artery.

Arterial lines can be placed in various arteries like the femoral, brachial and radial arteries. These lines are inserted via a surgical procedure to monitor the patient's blood pressure. Arterial lines can also be used to obtain frequent blood samples.

(95) (D) All of the above.

The nurse should be aware of the potential complications of having a pacemaker. Complications include pneumothorax, hemothorax, perforation of the pacemaker lead and cardiac tamponade.

(96) (B) Interpretation of ECG.

When there is a problem with the patient's ECG, the nurse has to interpret the ECG and decide on the next course of action.

(97) (D) All of the above.

The nurse should be able to explain how the disease process began. Patients should be told about the risk factors predisposing them to the disease. Nurses should inform patients about factors that can be changed and reduce the chances of developing the illness. The signs and symptoms of the disease should be explained to the patients so they can report to the doctor if they see any.

(98) (D) B and C.

Illness management begins with educating the patient about acute and chronic conditions. The education of patients includes information about the pathophysiology of the disease condition.

(99) (D) Arrhythmias.

Arrhythmias are mostly seen in hyperkalemia. Hypernatremia is an elevation of the sodium level above the usual standard. Hypernatremia can arise from several illnesses and conditions like diabetes insipidus, diarrhea, vomiting and Cushing's syndrome. Features of hypernatremia include thirst, agitation, restlessness and confusion.

(100) (C) An elderly patient with heart failure.

An elderly patient with heart failure has the most risk of developing bed sores because of reduced tissue perfusion and reduced mobility.

(101) (B) Observation of the patient for signs of immobility.

The first step in the evaluation of the patient for immobility begins with observation. Observation can reveal mobility issues that the patient might not be aware of.

(102) (C) Assess the patient using the CAGE questionnaire.

The best line of action is to assess the patient using the CAGE questionnaire to assess dependency.

(103) (D) Dietary modification.

Dietary modification is not a modality in the nonpharmacological management of pain. Nonpharmacological modalities include arts, music, companionship, massage, counseling, exercise and drama.

(104) (B) Hearing assessment.

Aspirin, gentamicin and hydrochlorothiazide are known to have adverse effects of ototoxicity. Hence a hearing assessment is the most appropriate evaluation in this case.

(105) (D) Polydipsia.

Polydipsia is not a primary urinary complaint.

(106) (D) Use of a smaller-sized urinary catheter to prevent pain and discomfort.

An appropriate-sized urethral catheter based on the age or size of the phallus should be used to prevent urine leakage if too small and urethral injury or discomfort if too large. Pain and discomfort during catheterization are minimized by anesthetizing the urethra with the passage of local anesthetic lidocaine gel.

(107) (A) Overhead trapeze bar.

An overhead trapeze bar is the best device as the patient's pelvic mobilization is limited to prevent further injury.

(108) (B) Intake of high glucose content meal.

Intake of high glucose meals will exacerbate dumping syndrome.

(109) (C) Hypocalcemia.

Hypocalcemia is unlikely to induce this state in the preterm neonate compared to the other above diagnoses. It should, however, be noted that hypocalcemia is a common problem of preterm neonates.

(110) (A) Pulmonary fibrosis.

Pulmonary fibrosis is not an anticipated respiratory complication of prolonged immobilization. Respiratory complications of prolonged immobilization include respiratory infections, atelectasis, hypostatic pneumonia, shallow respiration and decreased respiratory movement.

(111) (B) Neurological.

The neurological system is unlikely to be affected by prolonged immobilization. Systems commonly affected in prolonged immobilization include the integumentary system, pressure sores; musculoskeletal system, muscle atrophy; gastrointestinal system, constipation; and urinary system, urine stasis and infection.

(112) (D) All of the above.

She wants more drugs, which is drug-seeking behavior and is exhibiting withdrawal symptoms when she does not take her drugs, pointing to physical dependence.

(113) (B) High pain threshold.

Risk factors for substance abuse include a low pain threshold, several failed attempts at suicide, a high tendency to take risks, a high tendency to self-medicate and a concurrent mental disorder.

(114) (C) Prevention of falls.

Some things to be considered include achieving sobriety, participation in therapy and response to medications. Prevention of falls is not a factor that is considered when evaluating a treatment plan.

(115) (C) Displacement.

Displacement is a coping mechanism in which a client transfers anger, aggression or feelings of frustration at one person onto another person or object. In the question, the woman has transferred her anger and frustration at her baby's death onto her husband and friend as a way of coping with the fact that her baby died while she was not around.

(116) (B) Place her on observation.

Any threats of suicide or violence should not be handled lightly. The patient should be constantly observed, and restraints can be used if necessary.

(117) (A) Apologize for making her uncomfortable and ask what the gesture means to her.

A nurse must respect all cultures as long as it does not harm the client or other clients.

(118) (D) All of the above.

Patients might have psychological needs which can be diverse. They might battle with confusion, sleep disturbances and depression.

(119) (C) Authoritarian.

Some families operate in an authoritarian structure where the leader makes all the decisions with little or no room for deliberation among family members. Others run a democratic structure where all family members can deliberate on decisions to be made. Some other families run a laissez-faire leadership where individuals within the family unit are left to make their own decisions while the leaders support and provide the needed resources.

(120) (D) Anna's phases.

Grief models include Sander's phases of bereavement, which involve shock, awareness of loss, conservation, withdrawal, healing or turning point and renewal. Worden's four tasks of mourning include accepting the loss, coping with the loss, altering the environment to cope with the loss and resuming a healthy life. Engel's stages of grieving involve shock and disbelief, developing awareness, restitution, resolution of the loss, idealization and outcome.

(121) (C) Possible non-adherence to the treatment plan.

Some of the parameters to look out for in evaluating a client's adherence include the participation of the client in the plan or not, previous experiences where a similar treatment plan did not work, lack of insight of the client, denial, self-efficacy, internal locus of control and side effects of the plan.

(122) (D) Nonjudgmental disposition.

Nursing care for patients with alterations or perception loss must be done in a nonjudgmental manner, no matter what the clients say or the behaviors they display.

(123) (D) All of the above.

For nurses to effectively manage stress, they must be able to recognize nonverbal cues and respond appropriately. Using Hans Selye's general adaptation theory, some of the cues from the alarm stage are pupil dilation, increased heart rate, respiratory rate, glucose consumption, cardiac output and increased adrenaline and cortisol levels with attendant manifestations. The resistance stage is marked by increased cardiac output and a maintained respiratory rate and blood pressure increase. The third stage is exhaustion. Other signs to look out for include loss of consciousness, hyperglycemia and hypoglycemia.

(124) (A) Restating, paraphrasing, reflecting.

Restating involves repeating exactly what the client said to clarify what was said. Reflecting involves a reflection of what the client is conveying beyond the words that are said. Paraphrasing involves a nurse saying what they understood from what the client said in their own words.


(125) (D) None of the above.

Compatible drugs can be mixed in the same syringe, and not all drugs have drug-drug interactions.


(126) (A) Administer both separately.

Oil and water don't mix, so a colloid is formed, so this makes B wrong. Option C was not part of the question as the question was specifically intramuscular.


(127) (C) All of the above.

Adverse drug reactions are classified into six types: dose-related (augmented), non-dose-related (bizarre), dose-related and time-related (chronic), time-related (delayed), withdrawal (end of use) and failure of therapy (failure).

(128) (D) Tachyphonia.

Tachyphonia is not a blood transfusion reaction. A blood transfusion reaction is characterized by fever, nausea, anxiety, chills, warm, flushed skin and other symptoms.


(129) (C) Grouping and crossmatching.

Blood grouping and crossmatching should be done to ensure compatibility between the whole blood donor and recipient.


(130) (D) Circulatory overload.

Hypertension, respiratory distress, tachycardia and bibasal crackles (pulmonary edema) are all signs and symptoms of circulatory overload. Patients with pulmonary embolism often have sudden onset shortness of breath, chest pain and sinus tachycardia as the most common ECG findings. Patients with transfusion reactions often present with itching, chills, urticaria and fever.


(131) (D) Inferior vena cava.

Central venous catheters are placed into the heart's right atrium via the superior vena cava. Central venous catheters can be introduced into the superior vena cava via a peripheral vein, as with a PICC, or via the subclavian or jugular vein. The inferior vena cava is not involved.

(132) (B) Venous ulcers.

Venous ulcers are complications commonly seen on IV catheters placed in the lower extremities. Central venous catheter insertion can cause complications such as infection, pneumothorax, hemothorax, thrombosis and embolism.

(133) (D) Erythema and tenderness.

This signifies an inflammatory response that may be due to an infection.

(134) (A) Drug therapy in pediatrics.

Pediatric patients require especially accurate dosing due to their smaller size and the way their bodies metabolize medications. Small deviations from the appropriate dose can result in either therapeutic failure or toxicity. Therefore, you should adjust doses based on the child's weight and sometimes the child's body surface area.

(135) (B) 1 pint.

One pint is equal to 16 ounces of fluid, and 1 ounce is equal to 30 ml. Therefore, 1 pint is equal to 16 x 30 = 480 ml. So, 500 ml is slightly more than 1 pint.

(136) (D) Oral route.

The oral route of drug administration is the most common, most accessible and most convenient for patients. It is usually the first choice, except when a patient cannot tolerate it or when swift action is needed, then the intravenous route can be considered.

(137) (D) None of the above.

The name of the medication, dose and expiration date should all be verified.

(138) (C) Hyperalimentation.

Total parenteral nutrition is most often used for patients who require complete bowel rest.

(139) (A) Complete bowel rest, negative nitrogen balance, serious medical illness or disease.

The main reasons for using total parenteral nutrition are complete bowel rest, negative nitrogen balance and serious medical illness or disease.

(140) (A) To deliver total parenteral nutrition.

The purpose of a hyperalimentation catheter is to deliver total parenteral nutrition.

(141) (B) Moderate to severe pain.

Opioids are used to treat moderate to severe pain.

(142) (A) Drowsiness, constipation and nausea.

The common side effects of opioid medications include drowsiness, constipation and nausea.

(143) (C) To minimize pain to a tolerable level.

The goal of pain management is to minimize pain to a tolerable level.

(144) (C) Lowered blood pressure.

Some of the potential risks of opioid medications include addiction, constipation and respiratory depression. Reduction in blood pressure is, however, not one of the risks of opioid use.

(145) (B) Use of opioids.

Opioids are used to manage moderate to severe pain.

(146) (B) Infections and phlebitis.

Common complications from intravenous infusion therapy include infections, phlebitis, fluid overload and hematoma.

(147) (D) To ensure successful blood transfusion.

Selecting an appropriate vein is important to ensure a successful blood transfusion. If a vein is not patent enough, the blood transfusion can be affected. If the vein is also not good enough, it can lead to the formation of a hematoma.

(148) (D) All of the above.

The ability to think critically is important for RNs because some patients are given pharmaceuticals for a short time for acute sickness. In contrast, others may take medications for a chronic health issue for an extended time. Prescription pharmaceuticals, over-the-counter medications, vitamins, supplements and alternative medications are examples of these medications.

(149) (C) Consequences of a drug that are expected.

The term "side effects" refers to all the consequences of a drug that are not the expected therapeutic impact of the medication. They are also known as adverse reactions or adverse effects.

(150) (C) Eye color.

Patients may respond differently due to factors such as age, health status, genetics and individual variability in drug metabolism. Eye color will not affect drug metabolism.

## Test 4: Questions

(1) Which of the following best represents the role of a nurse as an advocate?

(A) Providing physical care to patients

(B) Administering medications according to the prescribed dosage

(C) Educating patients about their health conditions and treatment options

(D) Maintaining accurate documentation of patient assessments

(2) Which of the following scenarios best demonstrates the nurse's advocacy role?

(A) Administering a medication without informing the patient about potential side effects

(B) Supporting a patient's decision to refuse a recommended surgical procedure

(C) Following a standardized care plan without questioning its appropriateness for the patient

(D) Documenting vital signs accurately and promptly in the patient's electronic health record

(3) A nurse is working as a case manager for a patient who recently underwent a total knee replacement surgery. Which of the following tasks is an essential responsibility of the nurse in the role of case management?

(A) Administering pain medication to the patient as needed

(B) Collaborating with the surgical team to plan the surgery

(C) Coordinating post-operative physical therapy sessions

(D) Documenting the patient's vital signs during the hospital stay


(4) A nurse is acting as a case manager for a patient with a chronic illness. The patient requires multiple healthcare services, including specialist consultations, laboratory tests, and home health visits. Which of the following best describes the role of the nurse in this case management role?

(A) Providing direct patient care during hospital stays

(B) Conducting research to improve healthcare outcomes for the patient population

(C) Coordinating and integrating healthcare services for the patient

(D) Developing evidence-based practice guidelines for the nursing staff

(5) A nurse is caring for a patient who is being discharged from the hospital and transitioning to home care. Which of the following actions demonstrates the nurse's role in promoting continuity of care?

(A) Providing discharge instructions and educating the patient about self-care measures

(B) Administering medications to the patient during the hospital stay

(C) Conducting research to improve healthcare outcomes for the patient population

(D) Assisting with the admission process for a newly admitted patient


(6) A nurse is involved in a multidisciplinary team caring for a patient with a complex health condition. Which of the following best describes the nurse's role in promoting continuity of care within the team?

(A) Collaborating with other healthcare professionals to develop a care plan for the patient

(B) Conducting research to improve healthcare outcomes for the patient population

(C) Coordinating the scheduling of healthcare appointments for the patient

(D) Administering medications to the patient during the hospital stay

(7) A registered nurse is assigned a patient who refuses to receive the flu vaccine due to personal beliefs. What is the most appropriate response by the nurse?

(A) Disregard the patient's beliefs and administer the vaccine to ensure their health.

(B) Discuss the patient's beliefs, provide information on the benefits and risks of the vaccine, and respect the patient's decision.

(C) Tell the patient they won't be treated in the hospital unless they agree to take the vaccine.

(D) Report the patient's refusal to public health authorities.

(8) A nurse on duty overhears a couple of colleagues discussing a patient's medical condition in the hospital cafeteria. How should the nurse respond according to the nursing code of ethics?

(A) Ignore the conversation since she is not directly involved.

(B) Join the conversation and provide her own insights on the patient's condition.

(C) Report the incident to the hospital management.

(D) Politely remind her colleagues about the importance of maintaining patient confidentiality.

(9) A nurse is using the hospital's Electronic Health Record (EHR) system and notices that some of a patient's vital signs have been entered incorrectly. What should the nurse do next?

(A) Ignore it, assuming another healthcare professional will correct the error.

(B) Correct the error, then report it to the individual who made the mistake.

(C) Delete the erroneous entry.

(D) Document the correct values, note the error, and inform a supervisor or the person responsible for data management.


(10) A registered nurse is educating a newly diagnosed diabetic patient about managing his condition. The patient asks if there's a mobile app that could help him track his blood sugar levels. Which of the following responses is most appropriate?

(A) "Yes, there are several useful apps available, but you should discuss them with your healthcare provider before using one to ensure it meets your specific needs."

(B) "No, you should avoid these apps as they are not accurate and reliable."

(C) "I'm not sure, I don't keep up with technology."

(D) "You should rely only on your healthcare provider's advice and not on any mobile apps."

(11) A nurse receives a phone call from a patient's family member asking for information about the patient's health status. What is the most appropriate action for the nurse to take?

(A) Share all the information about the patient's health status with the family member.

(B) Confirm the caller's identity and share only the information authorized by the patient.

(C) Share minimal information and suggest the caller speak directly with the patient.

(D) Decline to provide any information due to HIPAA regulations.

(12) A patient has expressed the wish to refuse a recommended treatment due to religious beliefs. The healthcare team believes the treatment is necessary for the patient's survival. What should the nurse do?

(A) Respect the patient's wishes and advocate for their decision.

(B) Try to persuade the patient to accept the treatment, disregarding the patient's religious beliefs.

(C) Administer the treatment anyway, as it is in the best interest of the patient.

(D) Ask the patient to leave the hospital since they're not complying with the recommended treatment.

(13) A nurse observes that the rate of urinary tract infections (UTIs) on her floor has been steadily increasing over the last three months. Which of the following should be the nurse's initial action?

(A) Suggest that all staff members on the floor need retraining in sterile catheterization technique.

(B) Conduct a literature review on the latest evidence-based practices to prevent UTIs.

(C) Change the type of catheters used in the unit.

(D) Perform a root cause analysis to identify potential reasons for the increase in UTIs.

(14) The hospital administration has introduced a new procedure aimed at reducing medication errors. As a part of the quality improvement process, what should the nurse do after the new procedure has been implemented?

(A) Assume the new procedure is working if no medication errors are reported.

(B) Immediately begin planning the next quality improvement initiative.

(C) Collect and analyze data to evaluate the impact of the new procedure on medication errors.

(D) Request for a raise since the workload has increased.

(15) A 65-year-old patient with diabetes mellitus is in for a routine check-up. The patient reports increasing feelings of sadness and mentions having lost interest in activities they usually enjoy. The nurse recognizes these symptoms as possible indicators of depression. What is the most appropriate action for the nurse to take?

(A) Reassure the patient that these feelings are normal and part of aging.

(B) Recommend the patient take up a new hobby to divert their attention.

(C) Refer the patient to a mental health professional for further assessment.

(D) Keep the information confidential and avoid discussing it further.


(16) A patient with terminal cancer is experiencing escalating pain despite the current treatment regimen. The patient's family has expressed distress about managing the patient's pain at home. What is the most appropriate referral for the nurse to make in this situation?

(A) Refer the family to a counselor to manage their distress.

(B) Refer the patient to a surgical consultant for a surgical intervention.

(C) Refer the patient and family to a palliative care specialist.

(D) Refer the patient to a physical therapist for pain management exercises.

(17) A nurse is providing discharge education to an elderly patient who lives alone and has a history of falls. Which of the following instructions would be the MOST effective in preventing future falls?

(A) "Try to stay in bed as much as possible to avoid falling."

(B) "Always wear non-skid socks at home."

(C) "Keep your home well-lit, remove tripping hazards, and consider installing grab bars in your bathroom."

(D) "Avoid drinking fluids to decrease the frequency of bathroom visits."

(18) A nurse is performing a home safety assessment for a family with a young child. What recommendation should the nurse make to prevent accidental poisoning in the home?

(A) Place cleaning supplies and medications on high shelves.

(B) Rely on child-resistant packaging for medications and household chemicals.

(C) Teach the child about the dangers of medications and household chemicals.

(D) Remove all cleaning supplies and medications from the home.

(19) A nurse is working in a hospital when a code red (fire) is announced. What is the FIRST action the nurse should take as part of the emergency response plan?

(A) Evacuate all patients.

(B) Try to extinguish the fire.

(C) Ensure all room doors are closed in the affected area.

(D) Call the local fire department.

(20) During a mass casualty incident, the emergency response plan calls for implementation of the triage system. A nurse finds a patient who is breathing rapidly (35 breaths per minute) and has a radial pulse but is unable to follow commands. How should this patient be categorized according to the START (Simple Triage and Rapid Treatment) system?

(A) Immediate (Red)

(B) Delayed (Yellow)

(C) Minor (Green)

(D) Expectant (Black)

(21) A nurse is about to assist a patient in moving from the bed to a chair. What ergonomic principle should the nurse apply to prevent injury to self and the patient?

(A) The nurse should lift the patient using the strength of their back.

(B) The nurse should lift the patient primarily using their upper body strength.

(C) The nurse should maintain a straight spine and use their leg strength while assisting the patient.

(D) The nurse should bend at the waist while lifting the patient.


(22) A nurse spends a significant amount of time charting on a computer each day. What ergonomic principle can the nurse apply to prevent work-related musculoskeletal disorders?

(A) The nurse should adjust the chair and computer so that the feet are flat on the floor, thighs are parallel to the floor, and the top of the screen is at eye level.

(B) The nurse should sit on a high stool without back support to promote good posture.

(C) The nurse should position the computer screen below eye level to prevent neck strain.

(D) The nurse should sit cross-legged on the chair for maximum comfort.

(23) A nurse is caring for a patient with tuberculosis. What type of personal protective equipment (PPE) is MOST appropriate for the nurse to use when entering the patient's room?

(A) A pair of gloves and a gown

(B) A standard surgical mask and gloves

(C) An N95 respirator mask and gloves

(D) A face shield and a gown

(24) After administering chemotherapy medication, a nurse has to dispose of the empty medication vial. How should the nurse handle this?

(A) Dispose of the vial in the regular trash.

(B) Rinse the vial and then dispose of it in the regular trash.

(C) Dispose of the vial in a sharps container.

(D) Send the vial back to the pharmacy for disposal.

(25) A nurse is conducting a home safety assessment for a family with a 2-year-old toddler. What recommendation should the nurse make to prevent injury?

(A) Store all cleaning supplies and medications in lower cabinets for easy access.

(B) Place safety gates at the top and bottom of stairs.

(C) Use soft, fluffy bedding in the toddler's crib to provide comfort.

(D) Leave small objects on low tables to teach the toddler not to touch.


(26) A nurse is providing home safety education to a family with an elderly adult who uses a walker. What suggestion should the nurse provide to help prevent falls?

(A) Arrange furniture to create wide walkways for easy movement.

(B) Install area rugs to provide a soft landing in case of falls.

(C) Encourage the elderly adult to walk barefoot for better grip.

(D) Keep frequently used items on high shelves to encourage mobility.

(27) A nurse accidentally gives a medication to the wrong patient. Upon realizing the mistake, the nurse notifies the healthcare provider, monitors the patient, and thankfully, the patient suffers no harm. What is the next MOST appropriate action the nurse should take?

(A) The nurse should keep the incident to themselves since the patient was not harmed.

(B) The nurse should inform the patient's family about the error.

(C) The nurse should document the incident in the patient's medical record.

(D) The nurse should complete an incident report as per the institution's protocol.

(28) While performing a routine check on a medical device, a nurse discovers it is malfunctioning. No patient was harmed, but the device poses a risk for future patient care. What should the nurse do FIRST?

(A) Continue to use the device, but be cautious.

(B) Fix the device themselves to avoid any delay in care.

(C) Report the malfunction to the appropriate authority and remove the device from use.

(D) Ignore the malfunction if no patient was harmed.

(29) A nurse is preparing to use a mechanical patient lift to transfer a patient from the bed to a chair. Which of the following actions should the nurse take to ensure safe use of the equipment?

(A) Check the lift for any visible damage and ensure it is in working order before using it.

(B) Use the lift alone to transfer the patient, even if the patient is large or agitated.

(C) Ignore the weight limit of the lift since it is designed to lift all patients.

(D) Hurry through the transfer process to reduce the patient's anxiety.

(30) A nurse is caring for a patient who is on a ventilator. The ventilator alarms indicating a high-pressure alarm. Which of the following actions should the nurse do FIRST?

(A) Silence the alarm and continue with other tasks.

(B) Check the patient's respiratory status and the ventilator circuit for possible causes.

(C) Increase the oxygen concentration on the ventilator to ensure the patient is getting enough oxygen.

(D) Call the respiratory therapist and wait for them to arrive.

(31) A nurse is working in a pediatric unit and notices an unfamiliar individual attempting to enter the unit. The individual does not have an identification badge visible. What is the nurse's BEST course of action?

(A) Allow the individual to enter but keep a close eye on them.

(B) Confront the individual and demand identification.

(C) Prevent the individual from entering and immediately inform security.

(D) Ignore the individual as it's not the nurse's job to monitor access.

(32) A nurse is working in a hospital when a "Code Silver" is announced, indicating a person with a weapon is in the building. What is the FIRST action the nurse should take as part of the hospital's security plan?

(A) Run to the nearest exit to ensure personal safety.

(B) Lock or barricade the doors, turn off the lights, and keep quiet.

(C) Go find the individual with the weapon and attempt to disarm them.

(D) Continue working as usual but stay alert to any unusual activity.

(33) A nurse is providing care to a group of patients. For which of the following patient-care activities should the nurse wear gloves as part of standard precautions?

(A) Taking a patient's blood pressure.

(B) Providing a back massage to a patient with intact skin.

(C) Assisting a patient with oral care.

(D) Discussing a care plan with a patient.


(34) A nurse has just finished drawing blood from a patient. The nurse has a needlestick injury when disposing of the needle. What should the nurse do FIRST?

(A) Wash the puncture site with soap and water.

(B) Ignore the incident since the patient is not known to have any infectious diseases.

(C) Apply a bandage to the puncture site without cleaning it.

(D) Immediately start post-exposure prophylaxis medication.

(35) A nurse is caring for an agitated patient who is at risk of removing their therapeutic devices. Which of the following actions should the nurse consider FIRST?

(A) Apply soft limb restraints immediately.

(B) Administer a sedative medication to calm the patient.

(C) Explore alternative, less restrictive interventions to prevent device removal.

(D) Ignore the patient's agitation, and continue with routine care.

(36) If a nurse must apply restraints to a patient, what guidelines should they follow according to best practices?

(A) Apply restraints as tightly as possible to prevent the patient from removing them.

(B) Check the restrained patient every 8 hours.

(C) Obtain a physician's order within 24 hours of applying restraints.

(D) Provide opportunities for range of motion and circulation checks at least every 2 hours.

(37) A nurse is assessing a newborn 12 hours after birth. The nurse notes that the newborn's skin appears yellow. What is the most appropriate action for the nurse to take?

(A) Ignore the finding as this is a normal newborn skin color.

(B) Immediately administer a vitamin K injection.

(C) Report the finding and suggest a bilirubin test.

(D) Start phototherapy immediately.


(38) A nurse is teaching a new mother about how to care for her newborn at home. Which of the following instructions should be included in the teaching?

(A) The baby should be put to sleep on his or her stomach.

(B) Newborns should be bathed daily.

(C) The baby's head should be turned to the side during sleep.

(D) Newborns should be fed only when they cry.

(39) A nurse is performing a developmental assessment on a 4-year-old child. Which of the following skills would the nurse EXPECT the child to be able to perform?

(A) Write complete sentences.

(B) Dress themselves without assistance.

(C) Ride a two-wheel bicycle.

(D) Tie their shoes.

(40) A nurse is providing anticipatory guidance to the parents of a 3-year-old child during a routine health visit. Which of the following statements should be INCLUDED in the teaching?

(A) "Your child should have stopped napping by now."

(B) "Your child should be eating the same foods as the rest of the family."

(C) "Your child should have all of their adult teeth by now."

(D) "Your child should be reading by now."

(41) A nurse is caring for a woman who gave birth 24 hours ago. The woman reports increased swelling and pain in her legs. What should the nurse do FIRST?

(A) Advise the woman to rest more and elevate her legs.

(B) Massage the woman's legs to increase blood flow.

(C) Assess the woman's legs for signs of a deep vein thrombosis (DVT).

(D) Dismiss the woman's concerns as normal postpartum swelling.

(42) A nurse is teaching a woman who gave birth three days ago about signs and symptoms to report to her healthcare provider. Which of the following should be INCLUDED in the teaching?

(A) Fever higher than 100.4°F (38°C).

(B) Pain that is not relieved by pain medication.

(C) Heavy vaginal bleeding that soaks a pad within an hour.

(D) All of the above.

(43) A nurse is caring for a patient who recently received a diagnosis of terminal cancer. The patient states, "I just can't believe this is happening to me." How should the nurse respond?

(A) "You're just in denial, which is a common response to such news."

(B) "I understand that you're feeling upset right now."

(C) "Don't worry, new treatments are being discovered every day."

(D) "You need to face the reality of your situation."

(44) A nurse is caring for a patient who recently had a stroke and is struggling with new physical limitations. The patient appears to be increasingly withdrawn and expresses feelings of hopelessness. What is the nurse's BEST course of action?

(A) Encourage the patient to "stay positive" about their situation.

(B) Refer the patient for a mental health evaluation.

(C) Tell the patient that their feelings are normal and they will go away with time.

(D) Ignore the patient's feelings because they are a common response to illness.

(45)  A pregnant patient tells you that her last menstrual period started on April 15, 2023. Using Naegele's rule, what would be her estimated due date?

(A) January 22, 2024

(B) January 8, 2024

(C) February 22, 2024

(D) February 8, 2024


(46) Which of the following statements regarding the calculation of the estimated date of delivery (EDD) is CORRECT?

(A) Naegele's rule is based on a 30-day menstrual cycle.

(B) Naegele's rule is based on a 28-day menstrual cycle.

(C) The EDD is typically at 38 weeks from the date of conception.

(D) The EDD is typically at 40 weeks from the date of the last menstrual period.

(47) A nurse is assessing a fetal heart rate (FHR) on a patient who is 32 weeks pregnant. Which of the following FHR would be within normal range for this gestational age?

(A) 80-90 bpm

(B) 100-110 bpm

(C) 110-120 bpm

(D) 120-160 bpm

(48) During a laboring patient's contraction, the nurse notes a temporary drop in the fetal heart rate below the baseline that recovers after the contraction. The fetal heart rate otherwise remains within the normal range. What is the nurse's BEST course of action?

(A) Administer oxygen immediately.

(B) Reposition the patient on her side.

(C) Prepare for an emergency Cesarean section.

(D) Continue monitoring, as this is likely a normal fetal heart rate pattern.

(49)  A pregnant patient comes to you for her first prenatal visit. She is unsure of her last menstrual period. Which of the following is the BEST way to estimate her gestational age?

(A) Ask her to recall the date of conception.

(B) Wait until the baby is born and then assess its maturity.

(C) Use an early ultrasound to estimate gestational age.

(D) Use the fundal height to estimate gestational age.


(50) A nurse is providing prenatal education to a group of first-time mothers. Which of the following statements should be INCLUDED in the teaching?

(A) "You only need to take prenatal vitamins in the first trimester."

(B) "Regular exercise during pregnancy can be beneficial, but always discuss with your healthcare provider first."

(C) "You should consume at least 500 extra calories daily, regardless of your pre-pregnancy weight."

(D) "If you feel fetal movements decrease, wait until your next appointment to report it."

(51)  A nurse is educating a pregnant client about warning signs during pregnancy. Which of the following should be INCLUDED in the teaching?

(A) Mild morning sickness is a cause for concern.

(B) Swelling of the hands and face should be reported immediately.

(C) Lower back pain is abnormal and should be reported.

(D) Increased urination is a danger sign.


(52)  A nurse is providing education to an antepartum client about dietary needs during pregnancy. Which of the following is accurate information?

(A) Pregnant women need to triple their protein intake.

(B) Iron supplementation is generally recommended to prevent anemia.

(C) An additional 2,000 calories per day are required during pregnancy.

(D) Pregnant women should avoid consuming any fats.

(53) A nurse is preparing discharge instructions for a postpartum patient. Which of the following information is ESSENTIAL to include?

(A) "You should resume sexual intercourse as soon as you feel ready."

(B) "You should immediately start a rigorous exercise routine to lose the baby weight."

(C) "You should report any signs of postpartum depression to your healthcare provider."

(D) "You should start taking your regular medications without consulting your healthcare provider."


(54) A nurse is providing discharge instructions to a postpartum patient who plans to breastfeed her baby. Which of the following should the nurse include?

(A) "You should supplement with formula until your milk comes in."

(B) "It's normal to have some pain and cracking of the nipples."

(C) "You should feed your baby every 4-6 hours, or when the baby seems hungry."

(D) "You should drink plenty of fluids and maintain a balanced diet."

(55)  A nurse is assessing a new mother's ability to care for her newborn. Which of the following observations would raise CONCERN?

(A) The mother positions the baby on her back to sleep.

(B) The mother is responsive to the baby's hunger cues.

(C) The mother handles the baby roughly when changing diapers.

(D) The mother supports the baby's head and neck when carrying the baby.


(56)  During a postpartum home visit, a nurse is evaluating a new father's ability to care for his newborn. Which of the following would indicate the father needs further teaching?

(A) The father feeds the baby when the baby shows signs of hunger, rather than on a strict schedule.

(B) The father tests the temperature of the formula on his wrist before feeding.

(C) The father places the baby face down to sleep.

(D) The father carefully supports the baby's head while picking the baby up.

(57) A 60-year-old male patient with a family history of colorectal cancer presents for a health screening. Considering his age and family history, which of the following screenings would be MOST appropriate for this patient?

(A) Annual prostate-specific antigen (PSA) test.

(B) Biennial mammogram.

(C) Colonoscopy every 10 years or sooner.

(D) Bone density scan.


(58)  A nurse is reviewing health screening recommendations for a 45-year-old woman with a BRCA gene mutation. What would be an appropriate recommendation for this patient?

(A) Routine mammograms starting at age 50.

(B) Routine mammograms starting now, and consider MRI.

(C) Pap smear every five years.

(D) Colonoscopy every 10 years.

(59)  A nurse is performing a health and risk assessment for a new patient. Which of the following information would be MOST important to collect?

(A) The patient's most recent vacation details.

(B) The patient's family history of diseases.

(C) The patient's favorite type of music.

(D) The patient's hobbies.


(60) A nurse is assessing a 40-year-old patient who smokes, has a sedentary lifestyle, and a family history of heart disease. The nurse identifies these as risk factors for which of the following?

(A) Alzheimer's disease.

(B) Rheumatoid arthritis.

(C) Cardiovascular disease.

(D) Psoriasis.

(61) A nurse is conducting a targeted screening assessment on a 55-year-old female patient with a sedentary lifestyle and a BMI of 30. Considering these risk factors, which of the following screenings should the nurse MOST strongly recommend?

(A) Baseline eye exam for glaucoma.

(B) Screening for Type 2 diabetes.

(C) Annual skin examination for skin cancer.

(D) Hearing test.


(62) A 65-year-old male patient who has been a heavy smoker for 45 years comes in for a check-up. What targeted screening assessment would be MOST appropriate for the nurse to recommend?

(A) Screening for osteoporosis.

(B) Screening for colorectal cancer.

(C) Low-dose computed tomography (CT) scan for lung cancer.

(D) Screening for prostate cancer.

(63) A nurse is conducting an initial patient interview. Which of the following techniques is MOST appropriate to use to encourage the patient to share information?

(A) Directing the conversation and keeping interruptions to a minimum.

(B) Frequently checking the nurse's watch during the interview.

(C) Using closed-ended questions that require yes or no answers.

(D) Showing empathy and maintaining eye contact during the conversation.


(64) A nurse is taking a client's medical history. Which of the following communication techniques will help the nurse gather the MOST accurate and complete information?

(A) Rushing the client to avoid taking up too much time.

(B) Using medical jargon to demonstrate knowledge and expertise.

(C) Giving the client time to answer and asking open-ended questions.

(D) Telling the client what they think the problem is based on the symptoms.

(65) A 35-year-old patient presents for a routine physical. The patient reports working long hours, eating mostly fast food, and having no time for exercise. The nurse recognizes these lifestyle practices as risk factors for which of the following?

(A) Osteoporosis.

(B) Type 2 diabetes.

(C) Glaucoma.

(D) Tinnitus.


(66) During a health assessment, a nurse finds that a 45-year-old male patient smokes a pack of cigarettes daily, drinks alcohol frequently, and has a family history of lung cancer. Which of the following health problems should the nurse be MOST concerned about in regard to this patient's lifestyle practices?

(A) Alzheimer's disease.

(B) Rheumatoid arthritis.

(C) Lung cancer.

(D) Psoriasis.

(67)  A nurse is educating a 45-year-old client who smokes and is trying to quit. Which of the following strategies should the nurse MOST strongly recommend?

(A) Going "cold turkey" and relying on willpower alone to quit.

(B) Using nicotine replacement therapy as part of a comprehensive quitting plan.

(C) Cutting back on cigarettes gradually without the use of any quitting aids.

(D) Switching to a different brand of cigarettes that has lower nicotine content.


(68) A nurse is counseling a client with a sedentary lifestyle and obesity. What advice should the nurse give to help this client reduce the risk of developing Type 2 diabetes?

(A) Encourage the client to spend more time on hobbies like reading and watching TV to reduce stress.

(B) Advise the client to begin a regular exercise routine and make dietary changes.

(C) Recommend the client drink at least eight glasses of fruit juice daily to increase vitamin intake.

(D) Suggest the client reduce the amount of water they drink to decrease fluid retention.

(69) A nurse is preparing to participate in a community health fair. Which of the following activities would be MOST effective in promoting health and preventing disease in the community?

(A) Handing out pamphlets on a wide variety of health topics without any interaction.

(B) Setting up a booth to provide free blood pressure screenings and education about hypertension.

(C) Offering discounted memberships to a local gym.

(D) Giving a lecture on the importance of advanced medical directives to a general audience.


(70) A nurse is conducting a workshop on diabetes management in a community with a high prevalence of diabetes. Which of the following strategies would be MOST effective in ensuring the community gets the maximum benefit from this education?

(A) Conducting the workshop in medical jargon to display professionalism.

(B) Including practical demonstrations of blood glucose monitoring and insulin administration.

(C) Delivering the entire workshop as a lecture with no room for questions.

(D) Limiting the workshop to only those who have been diagnosed with diabetes.

(71) A 28-year-old woman comes to the clinic interested in starting birth control. What is the MOST appropriate initial question for the nurse to ask?

(A) "Would you prefer a daily oral pill or an implanted device?"

(B) "Have you thought about when you might want to have children in the future?"

(C) "Are you currently sexually active?"

(D) "Have you discussed this decision with your partner?"


(72) During a health assessment, a nurse is discussing contraception with a 22-year-old female patient who is not currently sexually active. The patient expresses a desire to remain abstinent for personal reasons. How should the nurse proceed?

(A) Advise the patient to start using a contraceptive method anyway.

(B) Discuss the different types of contraceptives in detail to encourage the patient to change her mind.

(C) Respect the patient's personal choice and discuss the importance of regular gynecological exams.

(D) Encourage the patient to get a contraceptive implant to be on the safe side.

(73) A 36-year-old female client with a history of deep vein thrombosis (DVT) wants to use combined oral contraceptive pills. What should the nurse's response be?

(A) "This is a safe choice, go ahead."

(B) "You should consider another form of contraception."

(C) "You can use them, but you must stop smoking."

(D) "This is an excellent choice for your age group."


(74) A client who recently gave birth 6 weeks ago and is exclusively breastfeeding her infant is considering using progestin-only pills as a contraceptive method. What should the nurse's response be?

(A) "This is not recommended as it can reduce milk production."

(B) "This is a safe and effective method for you."

(C) "You should consider a different form of contraception as this will harm your baby."

(D) "This is not recommended because it increases the risk of DVT."

(75)  A couple comes to a clinic for a family planning consultation. They express a desire to have two children, spaced 3 years apart, starting in the next year. Based on this, which of the following would be an expected outcome of their family planning?

(A) The couple will begin trying to conceive immediately.

(B) The couple will use a reliable form of contraception until they are ready to conceive.

(C) The couple will remain abstinent until they are ready to conceive.

(D) The couple will have a child every year for the next two years.

(76) A client with polycystic ovary syndrome (PCOS) is seeking family planning advice. She wishes to start a family but has been struggling with irregular periods. An expected outcome for this client's family planning is:

(A) The client will conceive naturally without any assistance.

(B) The client will need to adopt because she cannot have biological children.

(C) The client may need medical assistance, such as fertility treatments, to conceive.

(D) The client will have to wait until her periods become regular to conceive.

(77) A community health nurse is visiting a 75-year-old client for a routine check-up. Which of the following signs could indicate that the client is socially isolated?

(A) The client's house is impeccably clean and well-organized.

(B) The client has meals delivered regularly by a local service.

(C) The client has lost weight and has an unkempt appearance.

(D) The client takes daily walks around the neighborhood.

(78) A nurse is assessing a client during a routine health check. Which of the following statements made by the client MOST indicates environmental isolation?

(A) "I don't have any family living nearby, they all moved out of state."

(B) "I have difficulty walking and can't leave my home very often."

(C) "I attend a local book club every week."

(D) "I get regular visits from my home health aide."

(79)  A client with chronic migraines is interested in trying homeopathic remedies. As a nurse, what is the MOST appropriate advice to give?

(A) "Homeopathic remedies are safe and should replace your current medication regimen."

(B) "You can try homeopathic remedies, but do not stop your current medications without consulting your healthcare provider."

(C) "Homeopathic remedies are not effective, so you should not try them."

(D) "Homeopathic remedies can only be used in conjunction with acupuncture."


(80) A patient asks a nurse about the concept of "like cures like" in homeopathy. The nurse knows that this concept means:

(A) The same type of food that causes illness can also be used to cure it.

(B) A substance that causes symptoms in a healthy person can potentially cure similar symptoms in a sick person.

(C) A substance that cures an illness in one person will cure the same illness in another person.

(D) Illnesses can be cured by exposure to similar illnesses.

(81) A nurse is discharging a client who has recently undergone a hip replacement surgery. Which of the following observations is MOST indicative that the client may struggle to manage care in the home environment?

(A) The client has a two-story home with bedrooms on the second floor.

(B). The client has a family member who has volunteered to stay with them for the first week after discharge.

(C) The client is eager to get home and start their recovery.

(D) The client has arranged for a home health aide to help them three days a week.

(82) A nurse is evaluating a diabetic patient's ability to manage their care at home. Which of the following would indicate that the patient might struggle with home care?

(A) The patient correctly demonstrates how to check their blood glucose levels.

(B) The patient asks multiple questions about their medication dosage.

(C) The patient has a chart where they have been tracking their meals and snacks.

(D) The patient seems confused when discussing the timing of their insulin doses.

(83) During a routine home visit, a nurse notices that an elderly client has several unexplained bruises and appears malnourished. The client's caregiver is evasive when questioned. What is the MOST appropriate action for the nurse to take?

(A) Contact the caregiver's employer to report suspected abuse.

(B) Report the suspicions of abuse to the local authority or designated adult protective services.

(C) Offer the client additional meals during visits.

(D) Discuss the bruises with the client in the presence of the caregiver.


(84) A nurse in the emergency department is treating a patient with multiple injuries who is accompanied by a partner who answers all the questions directed to the patient. The patient avoids eye contact and appears frightened. What is the nurse's BEST initial action?

(A) Separate the patient and the partner to interview the patient alone.

(B) Ask the partner to leave the room immediately.

(C) Directly ask the patient if their partner is hurting them.

(D) Notify the police about a possible domestic violence situation.

(85) Which of the following is a known risk factor for domestic abuse?

(A) The victim having a high level of education

(B) The abuser exhibiting controlling behavior

(C) The victim having a strong support network

(D) The abuser having a low level of alcohol consumption


(86) A nurse is evaluating potential risk factors for elder abuse. Which of the following situations could MOST likely increase the risk of elder abuse?

(A) The elderly person lives in a nursing home.

(B) The elderly person's son, who has a history of substance misuse, recently moved into the home.

(C) The elderly person has a weekly visit from a home health nurse.

(D) The elderly person has a legally appointed guardian.

(87) A nurse suspects that a client is a victim of domestic violence. The client has shared that she feels unsafe at home. What would be the MOST appropriate initial intervention for the nurse to plan?

(A) Encourage the client to confront the abuser.

(B) Develop a safety plan with the client.

(C) Suggest the client immediately leave the abuser.

(D) Advise the client to hide evidence of abuse to avoid further violence.


(88) A nurse is planning interventions for a child who is a suspected victim of abuse. Which of the following should be the nurse's HIGHEST priority?

(A) Ensure the child's immediate safety.

(B) Educate the parents about alternative discipline strategies.

(C) Teach the child to avoid behaviors that may provoke the abuse.

(D) Arrange for a psychological evaluation of the child.

(89) A nurse is caring for a client with chronic obstructive pulmonary disease (COPD). Which of the following alterations in body systems is MOST commonly associated with this disease?

(A) Impaired gas exchange

(B) Hyperactive bowel sounds

(C) Decreased intracranial pressure

(D) Hyperactive deep tendon reflexes

(90) A nurse is caring for a client with type 2 diabetes mellitus. The nurse knows that which of the following body system alterations is MOST common in this disease?

(A) Impaired digestion

(B) Impaired gas exchange

(C) Increased platelet aggregation

(D) Decreased cardiac output

(91) A nurse is reviewing lab results for a client admitted with dehydration. Which of the following lab findings is MOST consistent with this condition?

(A) Decreased serum sodium

(B) Increased hematocrit

(C) Decreased blood urea nitrogen (BUN)

(D) Decreased serum potassium


(92) A client with chronic kidney disease is at risk for which electrolyte imbalance?

(A) Hypocalcemia

(B) Hypokalemia

(C) Hyponatremia

(D) Hypophosphatemia

(93) A nurse is assessing a client with a diagnosis of left-sided heart failure. Which of the following clinical manifestations is primarily related to a decrease in cardiac output?

(A) Distended neck veins

(B) Crackles in the lungs

(C) Fatigue and weakness

(D) Peripheral edema


(94) A client is experiencing hypovolemic shock after a severe injury. Which of the following is an expected hemodynamic change?

(A) Increased cardiac output

(B) Increased systemic vascular resistance (SVR)

(C) Decreased central venous pressure (CVP)

(D) Decreased heart rate

(95) A nurse is educating a patient recently diagnosed with type 2 diabetes on illness management. Which of the following statements by the patient indicates a need for further teaching?

(A) "I will need to monitor my blood sugar levels regularly."

(B) "Exercise is not that important since I am on medication."

(C) "I will need to make some dietary changes to manage my condition."

(D) "Regular check-ups with my healthcare provider are important."


(96) A client with chronic obstructive pulmonary disease (COPD) is being discharged. The nurse instructs the client on illness management at home. Which of the following instructions is MOST important?

(A) Engage in vigorous exercise to build lung strength

(B) Use oxygen as prescribed by the doctor

(C) Take a double dose of bronchodilators if breathlessness increases

(D) Drink less fluid to avoid coughing

(97) A nurse is preparing a client for a magnetic resonance imaging (MRI) scan. Which of the following is MOST important to assess before the procedure?

(A) If the client has had a recent meal

(B) If the client is claustrophobic

(C) If the client has any metal implants or devices

(D) If the client has taken their daily medications

(98) A client's laboratory report shows a potassium level of 3.2 mEq/L. The nurse interprets this result as:

(A) Normal range

(B) Hyperkalemia

(C) Hypokalemia

(D) Hypocalcemia

(99) A client's laboratory report indicates a white blood cell (WBC) count of 12,000/mm^3. The nurse should interpret this finding as:

(A) Within the normal range

(B) Leukopenia

(C) Leukocytosis

(D) Neutropenia


(100) A client's lab results show a serum creatinine level of 2.1 mg/dL. How should the nurse interpret this finding?

(A) Within the normal range

(B) Indicative of renal impairment

(C) Sign of liver disease

(D) Sign of dehydration

(101) A nurse is reviewing the laboratory report of a patient and notes a platelet count of 90,000/uL. How should the nurse interpret this finding?

(A) Normal platelet count

(B) Thrombocytosis

(C) Thrombocytopenia

(D) Polycythemia

(102) The nurse is reviewing a client's laboratory results and notes a blood glucose level of 220 mg/dL. The nurse understands that this value indicates:

(A) Hypoglycemia

(B) Normal blood glucose level

(C) Hyperglycemia

(D) Normal fasting blood glucose level

(103) A client who underwent a laparoscopic cholecystectomy 24 hours ago is complaining of abdominal pain, bloating, and nausea. The nurse should be MOST concerned about:

(A) Postoperative infection

(B) Postoperative ileus

(C) Reaction to anesthesia

(D) Incisional hernia

(104) A client is admitted to the surgical unit following a total hip replacement. Which of the following signs would be MOST indicative of a potential postoperative complication?

(A) Moderate pain at the surgical site

(B) Inability to bear weight on the affected leg

(C) Swelling and warmth in the calf of the unaffected leg

(D) Mild disorientation due to anesthesia

(105) A nurse is preparing a client for a bronchoscopy. Which of the following is an appropriate nursing action in this case?

(A) Encourage the client to drink lots of fluids before the procedure

(B) Inform the client that they can eat normally right after the procedure

(C) Explain to the client that they might feel some discomfort during the procedure

(D) Assure the client that there is no need for sedation during the procedure


(106) A client is receiving peritoneal dialysis. Which of the following findings should the nurse report immediately?

(A) Clear, straw-colored outflow

(B) Cloudy outflow

(C) Weight loss after treatment

(D) Mild abdominal discomfort during treatment

(107) The nurse is preparing to administer a unit of packed red blood cells (PRBCs) to a client. Which of the following interventions is MOST important to prevent a transfusion reaction?

(A) Verify the client's identity with another nurse

(B) Infuse the blood product slowly over 4 hours

(C) Assess the client's vital signs every 15 minutes during the transfusion

(D) Warm the blood product to body temperature before administration


(108) A client who is receiving a blood transfusion complains of back pain, chills, and dyspnea. The nurse notes the client's temperature has increased by 1°C since the transfusion started. What should the nurse do FIRST?

(A) Administer an antipyretic to decrease the client's temperature

(B) Slow the rate of the blood transfusion

(C) Discontinue the blood transfusion

(D) Reassure the client that these are normal side effects of a blood transfusion

(109) The nurse is preparing to flush a client's central venous catheter (CVC). Which of the following is the best practice for this procedure?

(A) Use a 10 mL or larger syringe

(B) Use a 3 mL syringe

(C) Use a 5 mL syringe

(D) The size of the syringe doesn't matter

(110) Which of the following is a sign of potential infection in a patient with a central venous access device (CVAD)?

(A) Increased thirst

(B) Redness and swelling at the site

(C) Decreased pulse rate

(D) Increased urine output

(111) A nurse is teaching a client about home care for a peripherally inserted central catheter (PICC). Which statement by the client indicates a need for further teaching?

(A) "I will keep the dressing dry and clean."

(B) "I can remove the dressing and take a shower."

(C) "I should call my doctor if I have a fever or chills."

(D) "I will avoid lifting heavy items with the arm that has the PICC."


(112) Which of the following interventions should the nurse perform first when there is a suspected air embolism in a patient with a central venous access device?

(A) Administer oxygen

(B) Clamp the catheter

(C) Place the patient on the left side in the Trendelenburg position

(D) Notify the physician

(113) The doctor orders 200 mg of a medication for a patient. The medication is available in 100 mg/ml vials. How many milliliters should the nurse administer?

(A) 1 ml

(B) 2 ml

(C) 3 ml

(D) 4 ml

(114) The provider prescribes 500 mg of amoxicillin to be given orally. The medication is supplied in 250 mg/5 ml. How many milliliters will the nurse administer?

(A) 5 ml

(B) 10 ml

(C) 15 ml

(D) 20 ml

(115) A nurse is preparing to administer heparin 7500 units subcutaneously to a patient. The vial reads 10,000 units/ml. How many milliliters will the nurse draw up?

(A) 0.5 ml

(B) 0.75 ml

(C) 1 ml

(D) 1.25 ml

(116) A pediatric patient is ordered 8 mg/kg of drug X once daily. The child weighs 15 kg. How many milligrams will the child receive?

(A) 80 mg

(B) 100 mg

(C) 120 mg

(D) 150 mg

(117) A patient is prescribed a medication that should be given at 5 mg/kg/day divided into two doses. The patient weighs 70 kg. The medication comes in 250 mg tablets. How many tablets should the nurse administer for each dose?

(A) 1 tablet

(B) 2 tablets

(C) 3 tablets

(D) 4 tablets

(118) A nurse is preparing to administer a continuous IV infusion of Dopamine. The patient weighs 50 kg, and the physician has ordered a dose of 5 mcg/kg/min. The Dopamine is mixed as 400 mg in 250 ml of normal saline. How many milliliters per hour should the nurse set the IV pump to deliver?

(A) 4 ml/hour

(B) 8 ml/hour

(C) 16 ml/hour

(D) 32 ml/hour

(119) A patient's IV infusion pump is set to deliver 125 ml/hour of normal saline. The nurse on shift checks the IV bag at 2 PM and finds there are 750 ml remaining. If the IV pump continues to infuse at the same rate, at what time will the bag be empty?

(A) 8 PM

(B) 9 PM

(C) 10 PM

(D) 6 PM

(120) A patient has a peripheral IV site that is showing signs of phlebitis: redness, warmth, and a palpable venous cord. Which of the following actions should the nurse take first?

(A) Apply a warm compress to the area.

(B) Document the findings and continue to monitor the site.

(C) Discontinue the IV and prepare to start a new IV in a different site.

(D) Administer a prescribed analgesic for pain relief.

(121) A patient who has recently undergone abdominal surgery is prescribed morphine sulfate for post-operative pain management. What is the priority assessment the nurse should perform before administering this medication?

(A) Assess the patient's level of consciousness.

(B) Check the patient's blood pressure.

(C) Assess the patient's pain level.

(D) Check the patient's allergies.


(122) A patient with chronic pain is prescribed a long-acting opioid analgesic twice daily and a short-acting opioid analgesic for breakthrough pain. The patient tells the nurse they are still experiencing pain despite taking the prescribed medications. What is the most appropriate response by the nurse?

(A) "I will notify the doctor that your pain is not well controlled."

(B) "You should increase the dose of your long-acting opioid."

(C) "You should take more of your short-acting opioid."

(D) "Pain is a normal part of chronic conditions and you will have to learn to live with it."

(123) A patient has just started on total parenteral nutrition (TPN) via a central line. Which of the following laboratory results should the nurse closely monitor?

(A) Complete blood count (CBC)

(B) Hemoglobin and hematocrit

(C) Blood urea nitrogen (BUN) and creatinine

(D) Blood glucose and electrolytes

(124) The nurse is preparing to hang a new bag of total parenteral nutrition (TPN) for a patient, but notices that the solution is cloudy and there are visible particles. What is the most appropriate action by the nurse?

(A) Shake the bag to mix the solution.

(B) Hang the bag and monitor the patient closely.

(C) Discard the bag and prepare a new one.

(D) Call the pharmacy for clarification.

(125) A patient with a left-sided stroke is learning to walk with a cane. On which side should the patient use the cane?

(A) Left side

(B) Right side

(C) Either side, based on patient's comfort

(D) Neither side, the patient should use a walker instead

(126) A nurse is instructing a patient on the use of a walker. Which of the following instructions is appropriate?

(A) Move the walker ahead and then step to meet it.

(B) Move one leg ahead with the walker, then bring the other leg to meet it.

(C) Lift the walker, move forward, and then set the walker down.

(D) Always keep both hands on the walker when sitting down or standing up.


(127) A nurse is providing health education to a group of middle-aged adults about good sleep hygiene. Which of the following would the nurse include as a recommended practice?

(A) Engage in vigorous exercise just before bedtime.

(B) Use your bed for activities like reading, watching TV, and eating.

(C) Establish a consistent sleep schedule.

(D) Consume caffeinated beverages in the evening to help stay alert until bedtime.

(128) A patient reports difficulty sleeping. The nurse asks about the patient's bedtime routine and discovers the patient often works on a laptop in bed before trying to sleep. What advice should the nurse provide?

(A) Continue with the current routine, but try wearing a sleep mask.

(B) It's best to work in bed to conserve energy for sleep.

(C) Move work-related activities out of the bedroom to strengthen the association of the bed with sleep.

(D) Drink a glass of wine to induce drowsiness before sleep.


(129) A nurse is teaching a patient with severe rheumatoid arthritis about maintaining personal hygiene. Which of the following recommendations is most appropriate?

(A) Take hot baths as hot water is better at killing bacteria.

(B) Use adaptive equipment such as a long-handled sponge for bathing and a raised toilet seat for toileting.

(C) Avoid showering or bathing to limit the risk of falls.

(D) Complete all hygiene activities in the morning to conserve energy.

(130) A patient with dementia often refuses to brush their teeth and becomes agitated when assisted. What is the best approach for the nurse to take in promoting oral hygiene for this patient?

(A) Force the patient to brush their teeth for their own good.

(B) Ignore oral hygiene practices to avoid agitating the patient.

(C) Try different approaches such as flavored toothpaste or a toothbrush with a large grip.

(D) Let the patient use mouthwash only.


(131) A nurse is educating a client newly diagnosed with type 2 diabetes about nutrition management. Which of the following statements by the client indicates they understood the teaching?

(A) "I will need to eliminate all sugar from my diet."

(B) "I will have to eat the same amount of food at the same time every day."

(C) "I should balance my meals with proteins, fats, and carbohydrates."

(D) "I should aim to eat as little fat as possible."

(132) A nurse is assessing an elderly client's nutritional status. The nurse learns that the client has poor dentition and difficulty swallowing. Which of the following nutritional interventions would be most appropriate for this client?

(A) Encourage the client to consume more fresh fruits and raw vegetables.

(B) Advise the client to drink more fluids and less solid food.

(C) Suggest a diet consisting mainly of soft, easy-to-swallow foods and nutritional supplements.

(D) Recommend increasing protein intake by consuming more lean meats.


(133) A nurse is providing education on oral hydration to a client with recurrent kidney stones. Which of the following statements made by the client indicates an understanding of the teaching?

(A) "I should drink at least 2 liters of water per day."

(B) "I will need to limit my fluid intake to prevent kidney overload."

(C) "Drinking coffee and tea in abundance will help to flush out the stones."

(D) "Water is not as necessary as long as I am consuming other beverages."

(134) An elderly patient was admitted for dehydration. The nurse instructs the patient's family about the importance of oral hydration. Which statement by the family member indicates a need for further teaching?

(A) "We will encourage him to drink even if he says he's not thirsty."

(B) "Drinking more water can help prevent constipation."

(C) "We should avoid giving him too much water because it can cause water intoxication."

(D) "We should aim for him to drink about 8 cups of fluid a day."


(135) A nurse is educating a group of nursing students about non-pharmacological comfort interventions for a patient suffering from chronic lower back pain. Which of the following interventions should the nurse include in her teaching?

(A) Administering a regular dosage of pain medication around the clock

(B) Recommending deep tissue massage on the affected area daily

(C) Encouraging the patient to perform regular, guided exercises

(D) Advising the patient to remain in bed and limit physical activities

(136) A nurse is taking care of a patient who has been experiencing chronic pain due to rheumatoid arthritis. Which of the following non-pharmacological interventions would NOT be appropriate for this patient?

(A) Applying cold packs to the affected joints

(B) Guiding the patient in mindfulness-based stress reduction techniques

(C) Encouraging the patient to participate in high-impact aerobic exercises

(D) Instructing the patient on the use of Transcutaneous Electrical Nerve Stimulation (TENS)


(137) A patient has been on bed rest for two weeks due to a complicated surgical procedure. Which of the following complications is the patient most at risk for due to prolonged immobility?

(A) Hypertension

(B) Deep Vein Thrombosis (DVT)

(C) Hypothermia

(D) Hyperglycemia

(138) The nurse is caring for a patient who has been immobile for an extended period. Which nursing intervention is crucial to prevent a common complication of immobility?

(A) Frequent turning and repositioning

(B) Limiting fluid intake

(C) Encouraging carbohydrate-rich diet

(D) Administering sedatives to promote sleep

(139) A nurse is educating a client on the use of a walker. Which of the following instructions is most appropriate to ensure safety and effectiveness?

(A) "Push the walker forward before you step."

(B) "Carry the walker and then step forward."

(C) "Place all your weight on the walker as you step."

(D) "Step forward first, then move the walker."

(140) A nurse is caring for a patient who is learning to use a cane following a leg injury. The nurse observes that the patient is holding the cane in the right hand, even though the left leg is injured. What should the nurse advise?

(A) "Continue using the cane in your right hand."

(B) "Switch the cane to your left hand."

(C) "You can hold the cane in either hand, it doesn't matter."

(D) "Hold the cane with both hands for added support."

(141) A nurse is caring for a patient who recently underwent a major surgery. Which of the following is a physical stressor that the patient is most likely experiencing?

(A) Fear of the unknown

(B) Financial difficulties

(C) Pain from the surgical incision

(D) Anxiety about returning to work


(142) A registered nurse is educating a nursing student about physical stressors. The student asks for an example of a physical stressor. Which of the following should the registered nurse provide as an example?

(A) Extreme temperatures

(B) Loss of a loved one

(C) Job-related stress

(D) Social isolation

(143) A nurse is caring for a patient who has recently been diagnosed with a chronic illness. Which of the following is a psychological stressor that the patient is most likely experiencing?

(A) Nutritional deficits

(B) Noise from the hospital environment

(C) Anxiety about the future health condition

(D) Pain from the disease


(144) Which of the following scenarios best describes a psychological stressor?

(A) A patient suffering from discomfort due to a fractured leg.

(B) A patient feeling stressed about moving to a nursing home.

(C) A patient experiencing extreme cold due to malfunctioning heating system.

(D) A patient having difficulty eating due to loss of appetite.

(145) A nurse is caring for a client with recently diagnosed macular degeneration, which results in a loss of central vision. Which of the following nursing interventions is most appropriate for this client?

(A) Encouraging the client to use peripheral vision

(B) Encouraging the client to close one eye to see better

(C) Avoiding the use of glasses to help improve natural vision

(D) Dimming the lights in the room to reduce eye strain


(146) A nurse is preparing discharge instructions for a patient who has recently suffered a mild stroke, leading to cognitive alterations. Which of the following actions should the nurse consider for effective communication?

(A) Providing all the information at once to avoid repetition

(B) Using complex medical terms to fully describe the condition and care

(C) Breaking down information into smaller, manageable chunks

(D) Avoiding the use of visual aids as they can confuse the patient

(147) A nurse is caring for a patient with recently diagnosed hearing loss. Which of the following interventions should the nurse implement when communicating with this patient?

(A) Speak loudly and quickly

(B) Use only written communication

(C) Speak clearly while facing the patient

(D) Use a high-pitched voice

(148) A nurse is preparing discharge instructions for a client who has been fitted with a hearing aid for the first time. Which of the following instructions is most appropriate for the nurse to include?

(A) "You should wear the hearing aid only when you are having a conversation."

(B) "It's okay to adjust the volume to the maximum to hear better."

(C) "You should gradually increase the amount of time you wear the hearing aid each day."

(D) "Avoid cleaning the hearing aid to prevent damage."

(149) A nurse is caring for a patient who has recently lost a spouse. The patient reports feeling a profound sense of emptiness and states, "I just can't imagine life without him." Based on Kübler-Ross's stages of grief, this patient's feelings are most consistent with which stage?

(A) Denial

(B) Bargaining

(C) Depression

(D) Acceptance


(150) A nurse is caring for a client who is displaying signs of complicated grief following the death of a loved one. Which of the following interventions should the nurse suggest?

(A) Encourage the client to avoid talking about the deceased loved one to reduce emotional distress.

(B) Suggest that the client seek counseling or join a support group for individuals experiencing grief.

(C) Advise the client to quickly get rid of the deceased loved one's belongings to expedite the healing process.

(D) Recommend that the client suppress their feelings of sadness and focus on positive thoughts.

## Test 4: Answers and Explanations

(1) (C) Educating patients about their health conditions and treatment options

The role of a nurse as an advocate involves supporting and promoting the rights and interests of patients. Educating patients about their health conditions and treatment options empowers them to make informed decisions about their care and exercise their autonomy.

(2) (B) Supporting a patient's decision to refuse a recommended surgical procedure

Advocacy involves supporting and respecting the autonomy and choices of patients. In this scenario, the nurse acts as an advocate by respecting the patient's decision to refuse a recommended surgical procedure. Administering a medication without providing information about potential side effects undermines patient autonomy.

(3) (C) Coordinating post-operative physical therapy sessions

Case management involves the coordination and management of healthcare services for patients across different healthcare settings. In this scenario, coordinating post-operative physical therapy sessions is an essential responsibility of the nurse in the role of case management.

(4) (C) Coordinating and integrating healthcare services for the patient

In the role of case management, the nurse is responsible for coordinating and integrating healthcare services for the patient. This involves ensuring that the patient receives appropriate and timely care from various healthcare providers and services. Providing direct patient care during hospital stays, conducting research, and developing practice guidelines are important nursing responsibilities but do not directly align with the role of case management in this scenario.

(5) (A) Providing discharge instructions and educating the patient about self-care measures

Promoting continuity of care involves ensuring a smooth transition between different healthcare settings and maintaining a seamless flow of information and services. In this scenario, providing discharge instructions and educating the patient about self-care measures are essential actions that promote continuity of care.

(6) (A) Collaborating with other healthcare professionals to develop a care plan for the patient

Promoting continuity of care within a multidisciplinary team involves effective collaboration and communication among healthcare professionals to develop a comprehensive care plan for the patient. This ensures that all team members are aligned in their approach to patient care and that transitions between different providers are seamless.

(7) (B) Discuss the patient's beliefs, provide information on the benefits and risks of the vaccine, and respect the patient's decision.

Ethical practice in nursing revolves around respecting patient autonomy, which involves allowing patients to make informed decisions about their health. This includes respecting their beliefs and providing unbiased information to help them make informed decisions.

(8) (D) Politely remind her colleagues about the importance of maintaining patient confidentiality.

According to the American Nurses Association (ANA) Code of Ethics, nurses have a duty to protect patient privacy and confidentiality. In this situation, the most appropriate immediate action would be to remind her colleagues about this obligation.

(9) (D) Document the correct values, note the error, and inform a supervisor or the person responsible for data management.

It is the nurse's responsibility to ensure accurate and timely documentation in a patient's EHR. If an error is detected, the nurse should correct it by documenting the correct values, note the error, and inform a supervisor or the person responsible for data management.

(10) (A) "Yes, there are several useful apps available, but you should discuss them with your healthcare provider before using one to ensure it meets your specific needs."

There are numerous mobile applications available that can help patients manage their health, including those specifically designed for diabetes management. However, it is important that the patient discusses this with their healthcare provider to ensure the chosen app meets their specific needs, is reputable, and will be a useful adjunct to their care plan.

(11) (B) Confirm the caller's identity and share only the information authorized by the patient.

According to the Health Insurance Portability and Accountability Act (HIPAA), a healthcare provider can share a patient's health information with a family member or friend if the patient has given their consent. However, the information shared should be limited to what the person needs to know for their involvement in the patient's care or payment for care. The nurse must confirm the caller's identity and ensure the patient has authorized them to receive information.

(12) (A) Respect the patient's wishes and advocate for their decision.

Nurses are obligated to respect patient autonomy, which includes their right to refuse treatment for personal, cultural, or religious reasons. While it may be challenging when a patient's decision might lead to harm or death, the nurse's role is to provide unbiased information, support the patient in understanding the implications of their decisions, and advocate for their rights.

(13) (D) Perform a root cause analysis to identify potential reasons for the increase in UTIs.

Quality improvement often begins with identifying a problem and conducting a root cause analysis to understand the underlying factors contributing to the issue. It is only after this analysis that appropriate interventions can be identified.

(14) (C) Collect and analyze data to evaluate the impact of the new procedure on medication errors.

Quality improvement is a continuous process, and evaluation is an essential step. After implementing a new procedure or policy, it's crucial to collect and analyze data to determine its effectiveness.

(15) (C) Refer the patient to a mental health professional for further assessment.

The patient's reported symptoms are consistent with depression, a serious condition that requires appropriate treatment. It is important for the nurse to refer the patient to a mental health professional for a comprehensive assessment.

(16) (C) Refer the patient and family to a palliative care specialist.

In this situation, referral to a palliative care specialist would be most appropriate. Palliative care professionals specialize in managing symptoms, including pain, in patients with serious illnesses. They also provide support to families managing these illnesses at home.

(17) (C) "Keep your home well-lit, remove tripping hazards, and consider installing grab bars in your bathroom."

Maintaining a safe environment is crucial in preventing falls among the elderly. Keeping the home well-lit can prevent falls related to poor visibility, removing hazards like rugs or clutter can reduce tripping, and grab bars can provide support in areas where falls are common, such as the bathroom.

(18) (A) Place cleaning supplies and medications on high shelves.

To prevent accidental poisoning, potentially harmful substances like cleaning supplies and medications should be stored out of the reach of children.

(19) (C) Ensure all room doors are closed in the affected area.

The RACE (Rescue, Alarm, Confine, Extinguish) acronym is commonly used to remember the steps to take in a fire situation. The first step is to Rescue anyone in immediate danger if it can be done safely. However, in most hospital settings, the announcement of a code red often means the fire is not in the immediate vicinity of the nurse or their patients. In such a scenario, the next step is to Alarm, which is often done automatically in hospital settings, and then Confine the fire. Confine, in this context, involves closing doors to prevent smoke and fire from spreading.

(20) (A) Immediate (Red)

According to the START system, a patient who breathes more than 30 times per minute, has a weak or absent radial pulse, or is unable to follow commands is categorized as Immediate (Red), indicating they require immediate medical attention.

(21) (C) The nurse should maintain a straight spine and use their leg strength while assisting the patient.

The principles of safe patient handling and movement emphasize using leg strength rather than back strength to prevent back injury. Keeping the spine straight helps maintain alignment and minimize strain.

(22) (A) The nurse should adjust the chair and computer so that the feet are flat on the floor, thighs are parallel to the floor, and the top of the screen is at eye level.

According to ergonomic principles, the chair and workstation should be adjusted so that the feet are flat on the floor, thighs are parallel to the floor, and the top of the screen is at eye level. This helps to prevent strain on the back, neck, and eyes.

(23) (C) An N95 respirator mask and gloves

Tuberculosis is spread through airborne transmission. Therefore, when providing care for a patient with active tuberculosis, a nurse needs to wear an N95 respirator mask, which is designed to protect against airborne pathogens. Gloves should also be worn to avoid contact with potentially infectious material.

(24) (C) Dispose of the vial in a sharps container.

Chemotherapy medication is considered hazardous waste. After use, empty chemotherapy vials should be disposed of in a sharps container to prevent injury and exposure to any residual medication. It is not appropriate to dispose of the vial in regular trash, as this could expose others to hazardous waste.

(25) (B) Place safety gates at the top and bottom of stairs.

Installing safety gates at the top and bottom of stairs can prevent falls and is a common safety measure in homes with toddlers.

(26) (A) Arrange furniture to create wide walkways for easy movement.

Wide walkways allow for safer and easier navigation, especially for someone using a walker.

(27) (D) The nurse should complete an incident report as per the institution's protocol.

Even when a medication error does not result in harm, it is important to complete an incident report to ensure the event is formally recorded and can be analyzed to prevent similar occurrences in the future.

(28) (C) Report the malfunction to the appropriate authority and remove the device from use.

When a medical device is found to be malfunctioning, it's important to immediately report it to the appropriate authority within the institution and ensure the device is not used until it has been checked and fixed by a qualified professional.

(29) (A) Check the lift for any visible damage and ensure it is in working order before using it.

Ensuring the mechanical lift is not damaged and is functioning properly is critical to the safety of both the patient and the nurse.

(30) (B) Check the patient's respiratory status and the ventilator circuit for possible causes.

A high-pressure alarm on a ventilator could indicate a variety of issues including a kink in the ventilator tubing, secretions in the airway, or a worsening of the patient's respiratory status. The nurse should first check the patient's respiratory status to ensure they are okay, then assess the ventilator circuit for any obvious issues.

(31) (C) Prevent the individual from entering and immediately inform security.

Ensuring the security of patients, particularly vulnerable populations like children, is paramount. If an unfamiliar person attempts to enter a secure area without visible identification, the nurse should prevent their entry if safe to do so, and immediately inform security to properly handle the situation.

(32) (B) Lock or barricade the doors, turn off the lights, and keep quiet.

"Code Silver" is used in many healthcare settings to indicate the presence of a person with a weapon or a hostage situation. The correct immediate response should be to follow the "Run, Hide, Fight" protocol, which typically involves securing your immediate location by locking or barricading doors, turning off lights, and staying quiet.

(33) (C) Assisting a patient with oral care.

Gloves should be worn as part of standard precautions whenever there is a possibility of coming into contact with blood, body fluids (except sweat), non-intact skin, or mucous membranes. Assisting a patient with oral care involves potential contact with mucous membranes and therefore requires gloves.

(34) (A) Wash the puncture site with soap and water.

If a needlestick or other sharps injury occurs, the first step should be to wash the puncture site with soap and water immediately.

(35) (C) Explore alternative, less restrictive interventions to prevent device removal.

The nurse should always consider and attempt less restrictive interventions before resorting to restraints. This might include diversional activities, adjusting the environment, repositioning the patient, or seeking the assistance of a sitter or family member.

(36) (D) Provide opportunities for range of motion and circulation checks at least every 2 hours.

When restraints are used, they should never be applied too tightly as this can cause injury and compromise circulation. Restraint checks should be done more frequently than every 8 hours, ideally every 15 to 30 minutes for continuous observation of the patient's physical and mental status. A physician's order should be obtained as soon as possible, not within 24 hours, ideally before applying the restraints or immediately after in an emergency situation. Providing opportunities for range of motion and circulation checks at least every 2 hours helps to maintain circulation and prevent muscle atrophy.

(37) (C) Report the finding and suggest a bilirubin test.

Yellow skin in a newborn may indicate jaundice, which is often caused by elevated levels of bilirubin. While a certain level of jaundice can be normal in newborns, it's important to monitor bilirubin levels to prevent severe hyperbilirubinemia, which can cause permanent damage.

(38) (C) The baby's head should be turned to the side during sleep.

This is an important instruction to prevent the risk of sudden infant death syndrome (SIDS). The baby should not be put to sleep on his or her stomach, as this can increase the risk of SIDS; instead, the baby should be placed on his or her back. Newborns do not need to be bathed daily, and over-bathing can actually dry out their skin. Feeding a newborn only when they cry is not recommended, as newborns need frequent feeding and may not always cry when they're hungry. Instead, a newborn typically needs to be fed every 2 to 3 hours.

(39) (B) Dress themselves without assistance.

Typically, by age 4, many children can dress themselves without assistance, although they may still struggle with buttons and zippers.

(40) (B) "Your child should be eating the same foods as the rest of the family."

At age 3, children should typically be able to eat the same foods as the rest of the family, as long as the foods are cut into small, manageable pieces to prevent choking.

(41) (C) Assess the woman's legs for signs of a deep vein thrombosis (DVT).

Increased swelling and pain in the legs can be a sign of deep vein thrombosis (DVT), a potentially life-threatening condition that is more common in the postpartum period.

(42) (D) All of the above.

All of the above symptoms could indicate a serious postpartum complication. Fever could indicate an infection. Pain that is not relieved by medication could be a sign of a complication such as a uterine infection or a retained placental fragment. Heavy bleeding could be a sign of postpartum hemorrhage. It's important for women to report these symptoms to their healthcare provider promptly.

(43) (B) "I understand that you're feeling upset right now."

This response validates the patient's feelings and communicates empathy, which is a crucial aspect of providing psychosocial support.

(44) (B) Refer the patient for a mental health evaluation.

The patient's withdrawal and expressions of hopelessness could be signs of depression, a common occurrence after a stroke. The patient should be referred for a mental health evaluation to further assess these symptoms and determine the appropriate treatment.

(45) (A) January 22, 2024

Naegele's rule calculates the due date by adding one year, subtracting three months, and adding seven days to the first day of a woman's last menstrual period. So for this patient, adding one year would be April 15, 2024, subtracting three months would be January 15, 2024, and adding seven days would be January 22, 2024.

(46) (D) The EDD is typically at 40 weeks from the date of the last menstrual period.

Naegele's rule, the most commonly used method to estimate the due date, is based on a 28-day menstrual cycle (not 30), but it calculates the EDD as 40 weeks from the first day of the last menstrual period (not 38 weeks from the date of conception). Although conception usually happens about two weeks after the start of the last menstrual period, it's more practical to use the date of the last menstrual period to calculate the due date because it's usually a definite and known date.

(47) (D) 120-160 bpm

Normal fetal heart rate is generally between 120 and 160 beats per minute. Lower heart rates could indicate fetal distress or other complications. Although fetal heart rate can sometimes be higher or lower than this range, any significant deviations should be evaluated.

(48) (D) Continue monitoring, as this is likely a normal fetal heart rate pattern.

This is describing a normal pattern called an early deceleration, where the fetal heart rate slows during a contraction and then quickly returns to normal. This is usually caused by head compression and is not typically a sign of fetal distress. Therefore, continuing to monitor the situation is the most appropriate response.

(49) (C) Use an early ultrasound to estimate gestational age.

An early ultrasound, performed in the first trimester, is considered the most accurate way to estimate gestational age if the date of the last menstrual period is unknown. While some patients may be able to recall the date of conception, this is often not a reliable method.

(50) (B) "Regular exercise during pregnancy can be beneficial, but always discuss with your healthcare provider first."

Regular exercise can be beneficial during pregnancy, but it's important to discuss the type and amount of exercise with a healthcare provider because some activities may not be safe.

(51) (B) Swelling of the hands and face should be reported immediately.

Mild swelling of the lower extremities can be normal in pregnancy, but sudden or severe swelling of the hands and face could indicate preeclampsia, a serious condition that requires immediate medical attention.

(52) (B) Iron supplementation is generally recommended to prevent anemia.

Iron supplementation is generally recommended during pregnancy because of increased blood volume and to prevent iron-deficiency anemia. Pregnant women do not need to triple their protein intake; the recommendation is an additional 25 grams of protein per day. An additional 2,000 calories per day would be excessive; the recommendation is an additional 300-500 calories per day, depending on the stage of pregnancy. Pregnant women should not avoid all fats; healthy fats are an important part of a balanced diet and are needed for fetal development.

(53) (C) "You should report any signs of postpartum depression to your healthcare provider."

It's essential to educate postpartum patients about the signs of postpartum depression and the importance of seeking help if they experience these symptoms.

(54) (D) "You should drink plenty of fluids and maintain a balanced diet."

Adequate hydration and nutrition are important for breast milk production and overall maternal health. It's not generally necessary to supplement with formula until the milk comes in; in the early days, the baby gets colostrum, which is low in volume but high in antibodies and other beneficial compounds. Pain and cracking of the nipples can be a sign of poor latch or other breastfeeding issues and should be addressed, not dismissed as normal. Newborns typically need to feed more frequently than every 4-6 hours; the general recommendation is to feed on demand, which is usually about every 2-3 hours for breastfed newborns.

(55) (C) The mother handles the baby roughly when changing diapers.

Handling a baby roughly is a red flag that the mother may need more education or support to safely care for her newborn.

(56) (C) The father places the baby face down to sleep.

Infants should always be placed on their back to sleep, not face down, to reduce the risk of sudden infant death syndrome (SIDS).

(57) (C) Colonoscopy every 10 years or sooner.

According to the American Cancer Society, men and women with an average risk of colorectal cancer should start regular screenings at age 45. However, for someone with a family history of colorectal cancer, the recommendation may be to start screening earlier and/or more frequently, depending on the specifics of the family history.

(58) (B) Routine mammograms starting now, and consider MRI.

Women who carry a BRCA gene mutation have a higher risk of breast and ovarian cancer. For these women, it is often recommended to begin mammography earlier than the typical starting age of 40 or 50, and to consider additional screening methods such as breast MRI.

(59) (B) The patient's family history of diseases.

A patient's family history of diseases is crucial information as it can help the nurse understand the patient's risk factors for certain conditions, such as diabetes, heart disease, or cancer.

(60) (C) Cardiovascular disease.

Smoking, a sedentary lifestyle, and a family history of heart disease are all established risk factors for cardiovascular disease.

(61) (B) Screening for Type 2 diabetes.

This patient's sedentary lifestyle and high BMI are risk factors for Type 2 diabetes. Therefore, a diabetes screening would be an appropriate recommendation.

(62) (C) Low-dose computed tomography (CT) scan for lung cancer.

Given the patient's long history of heavy smoking, he is at a high risk for lung cancer. The US Preventive Services Task Force recommends annual screening for lung cancer with low-dose computed tomography (LDCT) in adults aged 50 to 80 years who have a 20 pack-year smoking history and currently smoke or have quit within the past 15 years.

(63) (D) Showing empathy and maintaining eye contact during the conversation.

Showing empathy and maintaining eye contact helps to build a rapport, showing the patient that the nurse is engaged and interested in what they are saying. This encourages the patient to be more open and share more information.

(64) (C) Giving the client time to answer and asking open-ended questions.

Giving the client time to answer and asking open-ended questions encourage the client to share more information, leading to a more accurate and complete medical history.

(65) (B) Type 2 diabetes.

Working long hours, consuming a fast-food diet, and lack of exercise are lifestyle risk factors associated with Type 2 diabetes. Sedentary behavior and poor diet can lead to obesity, which is a major risk factor for Type 2 diabetes.

(66) (C) Lung cancer.

This patient's lifestyle choices (smoking and frequent alcohol consumption), coupled with his family history, significantly increase his risk for lung cancer. While all the conditions listed can be serious, this patient's specific lifestyle practices and family history align most closely with risk factors for lung cancer.

(67) (B) Using nicotine replacement therapy as part of a comprehensive quitting plan.

Nicotine replacement therapy can be an effective tool for smoking cessation when used as part of a comprehensive quitting plan that may also include behavioral counseling and support.

(68) (B) Advise the client to begin a regular exercise routine and make dietary changes.

Regular exercise and a balanced diet can help with weight management and reduce the risk of Type 2 diabetes.

(69) (B) Setting up a booth to provide free blood pressure screenings and education about hypertension.

Providing free blood pressure screenings and education about hypertension actively engages community members, provides a valuable service, and educates people about a common and serious health issue.

(70) (B) Including practical demonstrations of blood glucose monitoring and insulin administration.

Providing practical demonstrations allows participants to learn through observation and provides a chance to practice skills, leading to better understanding and retention of information.

(71) (C) "Are you currently sexually active?"

While all the options are valid questions during a conversation about contraception, the nurse should first determine if the patient is currently sexually active. This question is crucial to understand the immediate need for contraception.

(72) (C) Respect the patient's personal choice and discuss the importance of regular gynecological exams.

The nurse should respect the patient's personal choice of abstinence and focus on other aspects of reproductive health, like the importance of regular gynecological exams.

(73) (B) "You should consider another form of contraception."

Combined oral contraceptive pills are contraindicated in women with a history of DVT due to the increased risk of thromboembolism.

(74) (B) "This is a safe and effective method for you."

Progestin-only pills are considered safe for breastfeeding mothers and do not affect milk production, making this a suitable method of contraception for this client.

(75) (B) The couple will use a reliable form of contraception until they are ready to conceive.

An expected outcome of the couple's family planning, given their expressed desire, would be that they would use a reliable form of contraception until they are ready to conceive next year.

(76) (C) The client may need medical assistance, such as fertility treatments, to conceive.

Women with PCOS often have irregular ovulation or do not ovulate at all, making it more difficult for them to conceive naturally. Therefore, an expected outcome for this client's family planning could be the need for medical assistance such as fertility treatments.

(77) (C) The client has lost weight and has an unkempt appearance.

Social isolation can lead to neglect of personal care, which could be indicated by weight loss and an unkempt appearance.

(78) (B) "I have difficulty walking and can't leave my home very often."

Environmental isolation could be indicated by the client's statement about having difficulty walking and not being able to leave home often. This physical limitation could restrict the client's ability to engage with the environment outside of their home.

(79) (B) "You can try homeopathic remedies, but do not stop your current medications without consulting your healthcare provider."

While homeopathic remedies may be beneficial for some people, it's important to note that they should not replace conventional treatments unless under the supervision of a healthcare provider. Encouraging the client to consult their healthcare provider before making any changes to their medication regimen is appropriate and safest advice.

(80) (B) A substance that causes symptoms in a healthy person can potentially cure similar symptoms in a sick person.

The principle of "like cures like" in homeopathy means that a substance that causes symptoms in a healthy person can potentially cure similar symptoms in a sick person.

(81) (A)  The client has a two-story home with bedrooms on the second floor.

A two-story home may pose difficulties for a client recovering from a hip replacement, particularly if necessary facilities like their bedroom and bathroom are on the second floor.

(82) (D) The patient seems confused when discussing the timing of their insulin doses.

Confusion about the timing of insulin doses could potentially lead to dangerous situations like hypoglycemia or hyperglycemia.

(83) (B) Report the suspicions of abuse to the local authority or designated adult protective services.

The nurse has an ethical and legal obligation to report suspected elder abuse to local authorities or adult protective services.

(84) (A) Separate the patient and the partner to interview the patient alone.

In suspected cases of domestic violence, the initial step should be to try to interview the patient alone to ensure their safety and enable them to speak freely.

(85) (B) The abuser exhibiting controlling behavior

Controlling behavior is a common trait in abusers and is a significant risk factor for domestic abuse.

(86) (B) The elderly person's son, who has a history of substance misuse, recently moved into the home.

Family members with a history of substance misuse living with an elderly person is a known risk factor for elder abuse.

(87) (B) Develop a safety plan with the client.

Developing a safety plan with the client is a crucial initial step in intervention planning. It will include steps the client can take to protect themselves when violence occurs and how to safely leave the situation if they choose to do so.

(88) (A) Ensure the child's immediate safety.

The highest priority is to ensure the child's immediate safety. If abuse is suspected, necessary steps need to be taken to protect the child, which may include notifying Child Protective Services.

(89) (A) Impaired gas exchange

COPD typically results in impaired gas exchange due to obstruction of the airways, destruction of the alveoli, and problems with the blood vessels in the lungs.

(90) (C)  Increased platelet aggregation

Individuals with type 2 diabetes mellitus are at an increased risk for vascular disease, in part due to increased platelet aggregation, which can lead to the formation of blood clots.

(91) (B) Increased hematocrit

Increased hematocrit can be a sign of dehydration. As the body loses fluid, the concentration of red blood cells in the blood (hematocrit) can become artificially high. Decreased serum sodium and decreased serum potassium would not typically be associated with dehydration, as these electrolytes can become concentrated in the blood with fluid loss. Decreased BUN is also not typically associated with dehydration; BUN can become elevated when the body is dehydrated.

(92) (A) Hypocalcemia

Clients with chronic kidney disease are at risk for hypocalcemia (low calcium levels). The kidneys play a critical role in maintaining calcium balance by converting vitamin D into its active form, which is necessary for calcium absorption. When the kidneys are not functioning properly, this conversion process is impaired, potentially leading to low levels of calcium in the blood.

(93) (C) Fatigue and weakness

Fatigue and weakness are primary indicators of decreased cardiac output, as the body's organs and tissues are not receiving enough oxygen and nutrients.

(94) (B) Increased systemic vascular resistance (SVR)

In response to hypovolemic shock, the body will attempt to compensate by constricting blood vessels to maintain blood pressure and perfusion to vital organs, leading to increased systemic vascular resistance (SVR).

(95) (B) "Exercise is not that important since I am on medication."

Regular physical activity is a crucial part of the management of type 2 diabetes. It can help lower blood glucose levels, reduce cardiovascular risk factors, contribute to weight loss, and improve well-being.

(96) (B) Use oxygen as prescribed by the doctor

Oxygen therapy, when prescribed, is important in COPD management to help maintain adequate blood oxygen levels. Vigorous exercise could exacerbate symptoms in a client with COPD; instead, moderate, regular exercise should be recommended.

(97) (C) If the client has any metal implants or devices

An MRI uses strong magnetic fields, and metal objects can be attracted to the magnet and cause injury. Furthermore, the MRI machine can potentially malfunction or distort the images if metal is present. Therefore, before the MRI, it is crucial to ascertain if the client has any metal implants, devices, or even smaller objects like piercings.

(98) (C) Hypokalemia

The normal blood potassium level is typically between 3.5 and 5.0 mEq/L. A level of 3.2 mEq/L is below this range, indicating hypokalemia, or low blood potassium.

(99) (C) Leukocytosis

The normal range for a WBC count is approximately 4,500 to 11,000 cells/mm^3. A count of 12,000/mm^3 is above this range, indicating leukocytosis, or a high white blood cell count. This may suggest an infection, inflammation, or other conditions that stimulate white blood cell production.

(100) (B)  Indicative of renal impairment

The normal range for serum creatinine is typically around 0.6 to 1.2 mg/dL in men and 0.5 to 1.1 mg/dL in women. A serum creatinine level of 2.1 mg/dL is above the normal range, indicating potential renal impairment or kidney disease. Creatinine is a waste product filtered by the kidneys, and its levels in the blood can rise when the kidneys aren't functioning well.

(101) (C) Thrombocytopenia

Normal platelet count ranges from approximately 150,000 to 450,000/uL. A count of 90,000/uL is below this range, suggesting thrombocytopenia or a low platelet count. This can increase the risk of bleeding and can be caused by several conditions, including certain medications, autoimmune diseases, or bone marrow disorders.

(102) (C) Hyperglycemia

Normal fasting blood glucose levels range between 70 and 100 mg/dL. A level of 220 mg/dL is significantly above this range, suggesting hyperglycemia or high blood sugar. This could be indicative of diabetes or another condition causing high blood sugar.

(103) (B) Postoperative ileus

Postoperative ileus is a common complication after abdominal surgery and is characterized by abdominal pain, bloating, and nausea. It occurs when the intestines slow down or stop moving, preventing the passage of food or stool.

(104) (C) Swelling and warmth in the calf of the unaffected leg

Swelling and warmth in the calf of the unaffected leg could be a sign of deep vein thrombosis (DVT), a serious complication that can occur after surgery due to immobility. This condition can lead to life-threatening complications if a clot dislodges and travels to the lungs.

(105) (C) Explain to the client that they might feel some discomfort during the procedure

During a bronchoscopy, a flexible tube is inserted through the nose or mouth to allow visualization of the airways. While the procedure is typically performed under sedation, patients might still feel some discomfort.

(106) (B) Cloudy outflow

Cloudy or turbid outflow can be an indication of peritonitis, an infection in the peritoneal cavity, which is a serious complication of peritoneal dialysis.

(107) (A) Verify the client's identity with another nurse

The most crucial step to prevent a blood transfusion reaction is to verify the client's identity and the blood product with another nurse. This ensures the right client is receiving the right blood product, as a mismatch can lead to serious, potentially fatal, transfusion reactions.

(108) (C) Discontinue the blood transfusion

The client's symptoms suggest a transfusion reaction, which can be life-threatening. The nurse should immediately stop the transfusion to prevent further complications. After stopping the transfusion, the nurse should notify the healthcare provider, return the blood product to the blood bank, and treat symptoms per institutional protocol.

(109) (C) Use a 10 mL or larger syringe

For flushing a CVC, a 10 mL or larger syringe should be used. Smaller syringes create higher pressure, which can damage the catheter or cause catheter rupture.

(110) (B) Redness and swelling at the site

Redness, swelling, warmth, or discharge at the site of the CVAD may indicate an infection. This should be reported immediately to the healthcare provider.

(111) (B) "I can remove the dressing and take a shower."

The client should not remove the dressing and expose the PICC line. Instead, they should keep the dressing dry, including when showering. If the dressing becomes wet, it should be changed immediately.

(112) (B) Clamp the catheter

If an air embolism is suspected, the nurse should first clamp the catheter to prevent further air from entering the vasculature. Following that, they should place the patient in the left lateral decubitus position and Trendelenburg position, which may help to trap air in the right atrium and prevent it from moving into the pulmonary circulation.

(113) (B) 2 ml

The medication is 100 mg/ml, so to administer 200 mg, the nurse would need to give 2 ml (200 mg ÷ 100 mg/ml = 2 ml).

(114) (B) 10 ml

Using a proportion to solve, if 250 mg equals 5 ml, then 500 mg would equal 10 ml.

(115) (B) 0.75 ml

The vial has 10,000 units in each ml, so 7500 units would be 0.75 ml (7500 units ÷ 10,000 units/ml = 0.75 ml).

(116) (D) 150 mg

Using the weight of the child (15 kg) and the dosage ordered (8 mg/kg), the total daily dose for this child would be 120 mg (8 mg/kg * 15 kg = 120 mg).

(117) (B) 2 tablets

First, calculate the total daily dose: 5 mg/kg/day * 70 kg = 350 mg/day. This should be divided into two doses, so each dose is 350 mg/day ÷ 2 = 175 mg/dose. Given that the medication comes in 250 mg tablets, the nurse will need to administer less than a full tablet for each dose. Since tablets generally cannot be split into more than halves, the nurse will need to administer the closest amount to the necessary dose without exceeding it, which would be one 250 mg tablet split in half. This equates to 125 mg, which is the closest one can get to 175 mg using these tablets. Therefore, the patient should receive 0.5 (half) of a tablet for each dose. However, given the choices, the most accurate would be 2 tablets, if we consider the total daily dosage that should be delivered (350 mg), which may be possible with a different form of the medication or a different administration schedule.

(118) (D) 32 ml/hour

First, calculate the total dose of Dopamine in micrograms: 400 mg * 1,000,000 mcg/mg = 400,000,000 mcg. This dose is diluted in 250 ml of normal saline, so the concentration of the solution is 400,000,000 mcg/250 ml = 1,600,000 mcg/ml. Next, calculate the patient's dose per minute: 5 mcg/kg/min * 50 kg = 250 mcg/min. To find the volume of the solution needed to deliver this dose, divide the patient's dose per minute by the concentration of the solution: 250 mcg/min ÷ 1,600,000 mcg/ml = 0.00015625 ml/min. To convert this to ml/hour, multiply by 60 min/hour: 0.00015625 ml/min * 60 min/hour = 9.375 ml/hour. Because IV pumps cannot deliver fractions of a milliliter, the nurse should round this to the nearest whole number, which would be 9 ml/hour. This isn't an option, so the closest provided answer would be 32 ml/hour, which indicates a misunderstanding in the calculations or possibly a need for a different concentration or delivery mechanism for the medication. The options provided may not correspond with the actual calculation result, indicating a potential error in the question design. Always ensure to double-check calculations and to follow the specifics of the order and the available medication form and concentration in real practice.

(119) (A) 8 PM

To find out when the IV bag will be empty, we first need to calculate how many hours it will take for the remaining volume in the bag to be infused at the current rate. The infusion rate is 125 ml/hour and there are 750 ml remaining in the bag, so 750 ml ÷ 125 ml/hour = 6 hours.

If the nurse checked the bag at 2 PM, and it will take 6 more hours for the bag to be empty, then the bag will be empty at 2 PM + 6 hours = 8 PM. So, the correct answer is A, 8 PM.

(120) (C) Discontinue the IV and prepare to start a new IV in a different site.

The correct action to take in response to signs of phlebitis at a peripheral IV site is to discontinue the IV. Phlebitis refers to inflammation of the vein, and can progress to more serious complications if not addressed promptly.

(121) (D) Check the patient's allergies.

While all the options mentioned are important considerations before administering medication, the priority is to check the patient's allergies. It's crucial to ensure the patient does not have an allergy to morphine sulfate, which could cause a severe allergic reaction.

(122) (A) "I will notify the doctor that your pain is not well controlled."

The most appropriate response by the nurse is to notify the prescribing provider that the patient's pain is not well controlled. Pain management should be individualized and based on ongoing assessments of the patient's reported pain and response to treatment. It's not within the nurse's scope of practice to advise a patient to increase the dose of their medication. It's also inappropriate and not therapeutic to tell the patient to learn to live with the pain.

(123) (D) Blood glucose and electrolytes

While all of the lab tests listed are important in the overall assessment of a patient's health, the priority for a patient on total parenteral nutrition (TPN) would be to monitor blood glucose levels and electrolytes. TPN is a high glucose solution that can cause hyperglycemia, particularly when it is first started or the rate is changed. The high concentration of nutrients can also affect electrolyte balance, so the nurse should closely monitor these levels.

(124) (C) Discard the bag and prepare a new one.

TPN should always be clear and free of visible particles. If the TPN solution is cloudy or has visible particles, it may indicate contamination or instability of the nutrients. The nurse should not administer this solution. The most appropriate action is to discard the bag and prepare a new one.

(125) (B) Right side

The cane should be held in the patient's right hand, opposite the affected side, to provide support and improve balance by widening the base of support. The cane helps compensate for the weakness on the left side by taking some of the weight off that side. The right arm can then help the left leg move forward during ambulation.

(126) (A) Move the walker ahead and then step to meet it.

When using a walker, the patient should first move the walker about one step ahead, then step forward to meet it, maintaining balance and stability. This method provides the most support. Moving one leg ahead with the walker, then bringing the other leg to meet it would not provide balanced support.

(127) (C) Establish a consistent sleep schedule.

Establishing a consistent sleep schedule helps regulate the body's clock and can help with falling asleep and waking up. Engaging in vigorous exercise just before bedtime can actually make it harder to fall asleep because it raises the heart rate. Using the bed for activities other than sleep or sex can confuse the body's association of the bed with sleep.

(128) (C) Move work-related activities out of the bedroom to strengthen the association of the bed with sleep.

According to sleep hygiene principles, it's best to strengthen the association of the bed with sleep by moving work-related activities out of the bedroom. Working in bed can stimulate the mind and make it harder to switch into sleep mode. Wearing a sleep mask may help with light interference, but it won't address the fundamental issue of working in bed.

(129) (B) Use adaptive equipment such as a long-handled sponge for bathing and a raised toilet seat for toileting.

Using adaptive equipment like a long-handled sponge and a raised toilet seat can enable a patient with severe rheumatoid arthritis to perform personal hygiene tasks more comfortably and independently.

(130) (C) Try different approaches such as flavored toothpaste or a toothbrush with a large grip.

Trying different approaches can be helpful in promoting oral hygiene for patients with dementia who resist traditional methods. Introducing flavored toothpaste or a toothbrush with a large grip might make the process more pleasant and manageable for the patient.

(131) (C) "I should balance my meals with proteins, fats, and carbohydrates."

For people with type 2 diabetes, a balanced diet including proteins, fats, and carbohydrates is essential. Managing carbohydrate intake, rather than eliminating it is generally a key focus in the diet of someone with diabetes. Eating the same amount of food at the same time every day can be a part of managing blood sugar levels, but it's not the only factor to consider.

(132) (C) Suggest a diet consisting mainly of soft, easy-to-swallow foods and nutritional supplements.

A diet consisting of soft, easy-to-swallow foods and nutritional supplements can help ensure the client receives necessary nutrients without the risk of choking or difficulty swallowing.

(133) (A) "I should drink at least 2 liters of water per day."

For someone with recurrent kidney stones, adequate hydration, particularly with water, is very important. This helps to dilute substances in the urine that lead to stone formation. At least 2 liters of water per day is often recommended, though the exact amount can vary depending on individual needs.

(134) (C) "We should avoid giving him too much water because it can cause water intoxication."

While it is theoretically possible to drink enough water to cause water intoxication (hyponatremia), this is very rare, especially compared to the risks of dehydration in elderly patients.

(135) (C) Encouraging the patient to perform regular, guided exercises

Non-pharmacological interventions are those that don't involve medication. Administering a regular dosage of pain medication is not a non-pharmacological intervention. Deep tissue massage could potentially exacerbate pain in a patient with chronic lower back pain, depending on the cause of the pain.

(136) (B) Encouraging the patient to participate in high-impact aerobic exercises

High-impact aerobic exercises can increase joint stress and exacerbate pain in patients with rheumatoid arthritis. Instead, low-impact exercises, such as swimming or biking, are often recommended for these patients.

(137) (B) Deep Vein Thrombosis (DVT)

Prolonged immobility significantly increases the risk of developing Deep Vein Thrombosis (DVT), which is a type of blood clot that generally occurs in the deep veins of the lower leg or thigh. It can be life-threatening if the clot breaks off and travels to the lungs, causing a pulmonary embolism.

(138) (A) Frequent turning and repositioning

Frequent turning and repositioning is the most crucial nursing intervention to prevent pressure ulcers (also known as bedsores), a common complication of immobility. When a patient is immobile, constant pressure on certain parts of the body can restrict blood flow and lead to the breakdown of skin and underlying tissues. Regularly turning and repositioning the patient can relieve this pressure and improve circulation to those areas.


(139) (A) "Push the walker forward before you step."

The most appropriate instruction is to "Push the walker forward before you step". The walker should be moved first, followed by a step forward, allowing the walker to bear the weight and offer stability.


(140) (A) "Continue using the cane in your right hand."

The patient should hold the cane in the hand opposite to the affected leg. This provides better support and balance as it allows the patient to distribute their weight more evenly between the cane and the uninjured leg when the injured leg is moved.

(141) (C) Pain from the surgical incision

Pain from the surgical incision is a physical stressor. It directly affects the body and can influence the patient's overall wellbeing. Fear of the unknown and anxiety about returning to work are examples of psychological stressors. Financial difficulties represent a socio-economic stressor.

(142) (A) Extreme temperatures

Extreme temperatures are considered a physical stressor because they cause physical discomfort and can potentially lead to harmful physiological responses, such as heatstroke or hypothermia. Loss of a loved one and social isolation are examples of emotional stressors, while job-related stress is an example of a psychological stressor.

(143) (C) Anxiety about the future health condition

Anxiety about the future health condition is a psychological stressor. It involves the patient's mental and emotional response to the diagnosis of the chronic illness. Nutritional deficits and pain from the disease are examples of physical stressors. Noise from the hospital environment could be considered an environmental stressor.

(144) (B) A patient feeling stressed about moving to a nursing home.

A patient feeling stressed about moving to a nursing home represents a psychological stressor. This situation involves feelings of fear, anxiety, and uncertainty, all of which can affect the individual's mental and emotional well-being.

(145) (A) Encouraging the client to use peripheral vision

Macular degeneration is a condition where the central part of the retina (the macula) deteriorates, leading to loss of central vision. Encouraging the client to use peripheral vision is the most appropriate strategy as this area of vision is often retained in macular degeneration.

(146) (C) Breaking down information into smaller, manageable chunks

When dealing with patients who have cognitive alterations, it's important to break down information into smaller, manageable chunks to facilitate comprehension.

(147) (C) Speak clearly while facing the patient

Option C is the best choice because speaking clearly while facing the patient allows the patient to read the nurse's lips and facial expressions, which can help facilitate understanding.

(148) (C)  "You should gradually increase the amount of time you wear the hearing aid each day."

For a new hearing aid user, it can be overwhelming to suddenly hear sounds at a level they are not used to. Therefore, it is recommended to gradually increase the amount of time the hearing aid is worn each day to allow for adjustment. Option A is not correct because, for maximum benefit, the hearing aid should be worn as much as possible, not just during conversations.

(149) (C) Depression

The patient's feelings of profound emptiness and difficulty imagining life without their spouse align with the depression stage of Kübler-Ross's stages of grief. This stage is characterized by feelings of sadness, regret, and often a sense of hopelessness. It is important for the nurse to support the patient through this difficult time, providing comfort and empathy.

(150) (B) Suggest that the client seek counseling or join a support group for individuals experiencing grief.

With complicated grief, a person has a prolonged or significantly difficult time moving forward after a loss. They may be stuck in the denial, anger, or depression stage of grief. Counseling or support groups can provide a safe and supportive environment for expressing feelings and learning coping strategies.

4500
7200
73

4500 Dim
7210 } Bçs
7210
2000
_____
20 600